Plant Names in Homeopathy

An annotated checklist of currently accepted names in common use

Plant Names in Homeopathy

An annotated checklist of currently accepted names in common use

Vilma Bharatan[1,2], Christopher J. Humphries[1]
& John R. Barnett[2]

[1]Department of Botany, The Natural History Museum, London SW7 5BD UK
[2]Plant Sciences, The University of Reading, Whiteknights, Reading RG6 6AS

[VB02]   2002

Natural History Museum, London

126pp

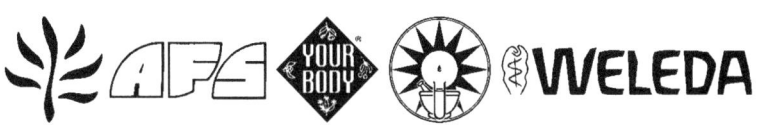

First published by The Natural History Museum,
Cromwell Road, London SW7 5BD
© The Natural History Museum, London, 2002
ISBN 0 565 09177 8

All rights reserved. No part of this publication may be transmitted in any form or by any means without prior permission from the British publisher.

A catalogue record for this book is available from the British library.

Written and edited by Vilma Bharatan, Christopher Humphries and John Barnett.
Page layout, design and setting by Diccon Alexander.
Printed by St Edmundsbury Press, Bury St. Edmunds.

Sponsorship: *AF & S Baker, Your Body Ltd, Helios Homeopathy Ltd & Weleda (UK) Ltd.*

Introduction:
Plant Names in Homeopathy; an annotated checklist of currently accepted names in common use

The 'plant' remedies used in homeopathy are mostly Angiosperms with some Gnetales, conifers, a few species of Lichen, brown and red algae, mosses and Ferns, and several species of Fungi. These 'remedies' have accumulated gradually during the past 200 years. As a result some are known by a variety of epithets, occasionally some of which are obscure, with names reaching back to the depths of time often with little justification with respect to a recognised code. In other words, the *Homeopathic Materiae Medicae* consists of both vernacular and common names, but mostly Latin names. However, at least half of the current names used in homeopathy need correcting with respect to the modern botanical code (ICBN, 2000).

In response to the problem this booklet provides a standard reference system for homeopathic practitioners, and other users of plant remedies by reconciling the old codes with the current *Botanical Code of Nomenclature*. The reasons for revision relate to the fact that the homeopathic *Materiae Medicae* have not adhered to a proscribed nomenclature standard, but various different codes largely of historical interest. This differs sharply from botanical practice where a whole set of agreed rules have been implemented for about a century. A revised list of remedies using currently accepted botanical names should provide an international standard that can be maintained and regularly updated in line with the revisions of the Botanical Code that takes place every six years.

Change in botanical nomenclature is an ongoing process as improvements to our understanding of plant taxonomy occur over time and classifications are reworked so as to express new systematic concepts. Generic and species epithets become modified for a variety of reasons. Homonyms, superfluous names, tautonyms, ambiguous names, rejected names, *nomina nuda*, and misidentifications are all in need of revision. Furthermore, taxonomic changes due to lumping or splitting of old species concepts and reassignment of misplaced taxa need to be accompanied by the appropriate changes of nomenclature. Using incorrect names leads to confusion and ambiguity, and in the worst-case scenario incorrectly identified plants could be used even in the preparation of homeopathic remedies.

Botanical Nomenclature

The *International Code of Botanical Nomenclature* (Saint Louis Code, ICBN, Greuter *et al.* 2000) provides for plants the nearest approximation to nomenclatural stability. It is the sixteenth edition and originated with the Vienna code of 1905 (See *Briquet in International code of Botanical nomenclature*, 1935). Modified and updated every six years (at the *International Botanical Congresses*) the code specifies how correct names for various groups of plants are determined and its operational core consists of a series of numbered rules or articles, some of which are supplemented by recommendations.

As more plants were discovered and described in the 18th and 19th centuries, divergent systems of nomenclature were then in use, which often resulted in the same plants being named more than once by different systematists working in ignorance of the publications of others. Although the priority principle was established by various authors prior to the Vienna Code, i.e. the oldest valid binominal name for each species was adopted, varying practice in different countries made it quite difficult to achieve stable nomenclature on a global scale. The Vienna code was thus formulated to overcome these problems.

Although a name is merely a convention, its main purpose is to act as a means of reference. Early plant names were simple nouns but as similarities and differences became realised, adjectives were applied to distinguish between species and other taxonomic groups. The noun gradually took on the role of generic name and adjectives became the specific epithets. As this use became more prevalent, a binominal (binomial) nomenclature was established. However, it was Linnaeus, the famous Swedish botanist, who consistently shortened the poly-nominal descriptions of species. He assigned each with two latinised words as a shorthand name, as in *Species Plantarum* (1753). Because Linnaeus described more than 9000 species of plants using binominal nomenclature, by convention the accepted starting date for the names of Ferns, Algae, Gymnosperms and Angiosperms is from *Species Plantarum* (Linnaeus, 1753). Mosses on the other hand start with Hedwig's *Species Muscorum* (1801). For most species of Fungi and Lichens, the starting date is *Species Plantarum*. However, as shown in article 13 of the Botanical Code of Nomenclature (2000; p25), names in the Uredinales, Ustilaginales and Gasteromycetes adopt Persoon's *Synopsis methodica fungorum* (1801) and names of other fungi adopted by Fries (*Systema mycologicum*, 1821) with the additional *Index* (1832) and *Elenchus fungorum* (volumes 1-2).

Taxonomic terminology

Following article 2 of the Code every plant belongs to a species as the fundamental unit of classification, which is placed into an indefinite number of higher ranks. The term taxon (plural - taxa) is a general term for any group of plants of any rank including genera, species and families. Thus, Solanaceae, *Atropa*, and *Atropa belladonna*, are the family, genus and species epithets for the homeopathic remedy, Belladonna.

The names of families are in Latin beginning with a capital letter and by convention ending with "*-aceae*". The only exceptions are some of the older names including Compositae (Asteraceae), Cruciferae (Brassicaceae), Gramineae (Poaceae), Guttiferae (Clusiaceae), Labiateae (Lamiaceae), Leguminosae (Fabaceae), Palmae (Arecaceae), and Umbelliferae (Apiaceae). Both versions of the family name can be used validly, but the Code recommends the use of "*-aceae*" family names for the sake of consistency.

To cater for infraspecific variation, ranks of subspecies (subsp.) and variety (var.) are used. Subsp. denotes one rank lower than a species and is used predominantly to indicate morphological differences often correlated with geographic distribution. Varieties (vars.) are ranks to denote consistent minor variants, e.g. based on flower colour and leaf length. For example, *Mikania amara* Willd. var. *guaco* (Bonpl.) Baker is a variety that differs from *Mikania amara* var. *amara*. It is important to note that in botanical nomenclature the authorities of the names or combinations are cited. Thus, for *Mikania amara* Willd. var. *guaco* (Bonpl.) Baker, Willd. is the author of the species, *M. amara*, and var. *guaco* is the varietal combination of Baker based on a new combination of the species *Mikania guaco* Bonpl.

Hybrids between two different species can be described as individual taxa, e.g. some authors consider the Seville or Bitter Orange *Citrus x aurantium* L., a hybrid. To recognise that an epithet is denoting a species hybrid a cross 'x' is placed at the beginning of the species epithet. Hybrids can also be represented by using both parental epithets connected with an 'x'. Therefore the parents of the Seville Orange could be represented by the following: *C. maxima* (Rumphius ex Burm.) Merr. × *C. reticulata* Blanco.

A species can have only one generic and one specific epithet, a precise point of reference. When a species is known by more than one name, then the first validly published name takes precedence over all later names, i.e. the rule of nomenclatural priority. All other names, even if apparently validly published, are reduced to synonymy. Synonyms exist for both nomenclatural or taxonomic reasons. Incorrectly formulated names not in compliance with the rules of nomenclature, together with unpublished names, are considered illegitimate and are no longer used. For synonyms that are possible homonyms (i.e. the same epithet used for different taxa) the author citation is especially helpful in distinguishing them, e.g. *Gelsemium sempervirens* has three homonyms, *Gelsemium sempervirens* (L.) W. T. Aiton (1811), *Gelsemium sempervirens* (L.) J. St.-Hil. (Feb-Apr 1805), and *Gelsemium sempervirens* (L.) Pers. (Apr-Jun 1805). All three names appear to be validly published, but the rule of priority establishes *Gelsemium sempervirens* (L.) J. St.-Hil. (1805) the currently accepted combination. The other two are illegitimate.

The checklist and database

Allocating correctly determined names to plants used in homeopathy according to the Code of Nomenclature, means that about 400 species require revision. Also, by taking into account most of the names published in the *Materiae Medicae* and the homeopathic Pharmacopoeias we calculate that approximately around 1700 names require consideration.

Plant remedies used in the *Complete Repertory* by Roger van Zandvoort provides the framework and guide for linking and associating all other names from their various sources. These sources are the *Materiae Medicae* and available editions of the American, French and German homeopathic pharmacopoeias (i.e. 1964, 1991, 1990 respectively). An important aspect of the new checklist is that every published authority has been checked from primary sources. We hope, therefore, that all citation errors have been corrected.

The checklist was compiled using a bespoke Microsoft Access™ database. The currently accepted species names are arranged alphabetically and relevant synonyms are presented, starting with basionyms[1], followed by other synonyms. All names conform to the rules of the Code with the authority, place and date of publication for each name given, and presented in that order. Abbreviated statements regarding status of the name follows directly after the bibliographic citation, e.g. *nom. nud.* (nomen nudum). Other statements include orthographic variants given in parenthesis, and unseen publications in curly brackets. An accepted name may have many

---

1 Article 33.3 of the coded notes that "A new combination, ...published on or after 1 January 1953 based on a previously and validly published name is not validly published unless its basionym (name-bringing or epithet-bringing synonym) or the replaced synonym (when a new name is proposed) is clearly indicated and a full and direct reference given to its author and place of valid publication of the basionym."

synonyms, but here, only those synonyms that have, or are used as homeopathic names, are included in this list. Other linked elements are family names, standard abbreviated remedy names in small bold capitals, letter codes, and where needed, additional information added as notes. These include common names, vernacular names, names peculiar to homeopathy and those names of different species that have been misidentified. Names that do not appear to have any nomenclatural status, even after exhaustive searches, are placed at the end of the checklist under 'untraced names'.

Design of the checklist and a detailed description of the elements of the text

Each current name is laid out in the form of an annotated checklist. Every entry consists of seven components: the accepted name with authorities and place and date of publication, family name, remedy abbreviation, letter codes for status within the homeopathic repertory and other sources, synonyms, and notes.

The accepted name
The accepted species name is printed in Roman boldface and arranged alphabetically.

Author names
This is an abbreviation of the name of the person or persons who first validly applied that name to the taxon. These are abbreviated to follow Brummitt & Powell (1992). For authorities not covered in Brummitt & Powell, abbreviations were formulated using their directives. Shared author names are connected by an ampersand, and for valid places of publication other than the proposing authority by *ex* or *in*. For new combinations, the original authority is placed in parenthesis and the second written after it. A citation within square brackets indicates a pre-Linnean author and auct. indicates many authors.

Publication citations
The title of the first publication in which the species name was validly published is given. The title is usually abbreviated and for titles of journals and serials, the B-P-H abbreviations (*Botanico-Periodicum-Huntianum,* Lawrence et al., 1968) and its supplement B-P-H/S (*Supplementum,* Bridson & Smith, 1991) are followed. For serials or journals not covered by B-P-H, abbreviations were formulated using B-P-H directives. For book titles, TL-2 abbreviations (*Taxonomic literature*, 2nd. ed., Stafleu & Cowan, 1976-88) and its *Supplements* (Stafleu & Mennega, 1992-) were used, but capitalizing all the words in the title. Further bibliographic details include edition number, series number, volume number, page number, plate and

figure numbers and the date of publication. Only the first page number is provided in all cases. Orthographic variations that are alternative spellings for a name are cited within quotation marks, e.g. *Eugenia chequen* Molina *U. S. Expl. Exped., Phan.* **536**. 1854, *"cheken"*.

Family names
The system of family names follows Brummitt & Powell (1992). See index for a complete list (Pages 98-120).

Remedy abbreviations
An abbreviation of the homeopathic plant remedy name used by the *Complete Repertory* (van Zandvoort, 1996) is written in small bold capital letters.

Letter codes for remedy names
The source of all the homeopathic plant names used in the checklist are listed using letter codes: Hn- Homeopathic name and Hs-Homeopathic synonym used by the *Materiae Medicae*; R-*Complete Repertory* name; A-*American pharmacopoeia*; F-*French pharmacopoeia* and G-*German pharmacopoeia*. When the initial list of homeopathic names was drawn, alternative names for each remedy were limited to two names per source.

Whenever cited the third or fourth lines of each entry contain the basionym or homotypic synonym. The basionym complete with author name and publication citation follows a similar format for the current names in the first line. Taxonomic or heterotypic synonyms are arranged in chronological order, with the author name and the title of the publication following the same format as that used by the accepted name. The nomenclatural status of each synonym is indicated by an abbreviated statement. This follows directly after the bibliographic citation. The glossary provides a full explanation for each statement.

Any additional information (e.g. incorrect usage) is included as notes as the last item of the entry. These include common names, vernacular names, names peculiar to homeopathy and those names of different species that have been wrongly applied.

Introduction

Glossary

& (Ampersand), used to link two author names. e.g. *Fabiana imbricata* Ruiz & Pav. auct. (latin, for auctorum), authors.

Binominal (or **binomial**), a phrase consisting of two words.

basionym, also known as homotypic or nomenclatural synonyms are based on the same type, resulting in a change of taxonomic position or rank. The specific epithet is retained, e.g., *Cactus grandiflorus* L. when transferred to the genus *Selenicereus* is called *Selenicereus grandiflorus* (L.) Britton & Rose. However *Arum dracunculus* L. when transferred to the genus *Dracunculus* was renamed *Dracunculus vulgaris* Schott, as the Linnaean epithet is a tautonym.

ex, (latin, from), used to connect the names of two authors, the second of which validly published a name proposed but not validly published by the first. E.g. in *Saccharomyces* cerevisiae Meyen ex E. C. Hansen, means that E. C. Hansen validly published the name which was originally proposed by, but unpublished by, Meyen.

f., (latin, filius) son.

homonym, identical names based on different types, thus duplicating a name previously and validly published.

in, (latin, in), used to connect the names of two persons, the second of which is the editor, or overall author, of a work in which the first was responsible for validly publishing a name. A citation such as *Micromeria chamissonis* Benth. in Greene indicates that Bentham validly published the name *Micromeria chamissonis* in a work edited or written by Greene.

incertae cedis (latin, of uncertain seat), of uncertain taxonomic position, e.g. *Cocculus indicus* Royle, Ill. Bot. Himal. Mts. 61. 1834, *incertae sedis*.

new combinations indicate a change in taxonomic position and/or rank of a species, but retains the species epithet. The original author is cited in parenthesis, followed by the name of the author who made the alteration. E.g. *Dieffenbachia seguine* (Jacq.) Schott indicates that this name published by Schott is based on the older name or basionym, *Arum seguine* Jacq. The name of the author of the basionym Jacq., is cited in parenthesis and precedes Schott, who made the alteration.

nom. ambig., (latin, *nomen ambiguum*), ambiguous name, a name used by different authors to mean different taxa, so it becomes a permanent source of confusion or error. E.g. *Crataegus oxyacantha* L. Sp. Pl. 1: 477. 1753, *nom. ambig.*

nom. illegit., (latin, *nomen illegitimum*), illegitimate name, a validly published name that does not conform to the rules of the botanical code. E.g. *Gelsemium sempervirens* (L.) Pers., Syn. Pl. 1: 267. Apr-Jun 1805. nom. illeg., not (L.) J. St.-Hil., Feb-Apr 1805.

nom. nud., (latin, *nomen nudum*), naked name; a name published without a description or diagnosis that satisfies the criteria for valid publication. E.g. *Jacaranda gualanday* Cortés Fl. Colombia. 99. 1897. *nom. nud.*

nom. rejic., (latin, *nomen rejiciendum*), a name formally rejected, usually in favour of another (conserved) name. E.g. *Lycopersicon lycopersicum* (L.) H. Karst., Deut. Fl. ed. 1. lief. 966. 1882, nom. rejic.

orthographic variants are different spellings for the same name. Only one variant of any name is treated as validly published, the form that appears in the original publication except as provided in Art. 60. The orthographic variation is given in parenthesis and follows on after the bibliographic citation. E.g. *Rauwolfia serpentina* (L.) Benth. ex Kurz Forest. Fl. Burma 2: 171. 1878. "*Rauvolfia*",

pre-Linnean authors are indicated in square brackets.. E.g. *Balsamum tolutanum* [C. Bauhin] L.

***p.p.* (*pro parte*)** latin for in part, used in citations to show that only a part of a taxon, as circumscribed by a previous author, is being referred to by the author.

sensu lato, in the broad sense.

tautonym, a name of a species in which the second word exactly repeats the generic name.

Annotated Checklist

Abelmoschus moschatus Medik., Malvenfam. 46. 1787.
    Malvaceae ABEL. Hn R A
    Hibiscus abelmoschus L., Sp. Pl. 1: 96. 1753. Hs
    Incorrect usage: *Alceae egyptiaceae* sensu Amer. Pharm., not Boiss.

Abies canadensis see *Tsuga Canadensis*

Abies mariana see *Picea mariana*

Abies nigra see *Picea mariana*

Abroma augusta see *Ambroma augusta*

Abrotanum see *Artemisia abrotanum*

Abrus precatorius L., Syst. Nat. ed. 12, 472. 1767.
    Fabaceae ABR. Hn R

Absinthium see *Artemisia absinthium*

Acalypha indica L., Sp. Pl. 2: 1003. 1753.
    Euphorbiaceae ACAL. Hn R G A

Acer negundo L., Sp. Pl. 2: 1056. 1753.
    Aceraceae NEG. R
    Negundium americanum DC. ex Loudon, Hort. Brit. 398. 1847. Hs
    Common homeopathic name: Negundo.

Achillea millefolium L., Sp. Pl. 2: 899. 1753.
    Asteraceae MILL. R G A F
    Incorrect usage: *Achillea myriophylli* sensu Amer. Pharm., not *Achillea myriophylla* Willd. Linnaeus (1749 p. 139) uses Millefolium (Hom. name) as the medicinal name for *Achillea millefolium*.

Achillea myriophylla see *Achillea millefolium*

Achillea myriophylli see *Achillea millefolium*

Achyranthes aspera L., Sp. Pl. 1: 204. 1753.
    Amaranthaceae ACHY-A. Hn R

Achyranthes calea see *Iresine calea*

Achyranthes repens see *Alternanthera repens*

Acokanthera schimperi (A. DC.) Benth. & Hook. f., Gen. Pl. 2: 696. 1873-76
    Apocynaceae CARI. R
    Carissa schimperi A. DC., Prodr. 8: 675. Mar 1844. Hn

Aconitum angustifolium see *Aconitum napellus*

Aconitum anthora L., Sp. Pl. 1: 532. 1753.
    Ranunculaceae ACON-A. Hn R

Aconitum ferox Wall. ex Ser., Mus. Helv. Bot. 1: 160. 1823.
Ranunculaceae ACON-F. Hn R

Aconitum lycoctonum L., Sp. Pl. 1: 532. 1753
Ranunculaceae ACON-L. Hn R
Aconitum telyphonum Rchb., Ill. Sp. Acon. Gen. pl. 54. 1825. Hs

Aconitum napellus L., Sp. Pl. 1: 532. 1753.
Ranunculaceae ACON. Hn R G A F
Aconitum vulgare DC., Syst. Nat. 1: 371. 1817, incertae sedis. A
Aconitum angustifolium Bernh. ex Rchb., Uebers. Aconitum. 29. 1819, incertae sedis. A

Aconitum neomontanum see *Aconitum x cammarum*

Aconitum septentrionale Koelle, Spic. Observ. Aconit. 22. 1787.
Ranunculaceae ACON-S.
Aconitum "septentrionalis" (Comp. Rep.) is an orthographic variant.

Aconitum septentrionalis see *Aconitum septentrionale*

Aconitum stoerkianum see *Aconitum x cammarum*

Aconitum telyphonum see *Aconitum lycoctonum*

Aconitum vulgare see *Aconitum napellus*

Aconitum x cammarum L., Sp. Pl. ed. 2, 1: 751. 1762.
Ranunculaceae ACON-C. Hn R
Aconitum stoerkianum Rchb., Uebers. Aconitum. 49. 1819. Hs
Aconitum neomontanum Willd., Willd., Sp. Pl. 2(2): 1236. 1799. Hs

Actaea racemosa L., Sp. Pl. 1: 504. 1753.
Ranunculaceae CIMIC. Hs
Cimicifuga racemosa (L.) Nutt., Gen. N. Amer. Pl. 2: 15. 1818. Hn R G A F

Actaea spicata L., Sp. Pl. 1: 504. 1753.
Ranunculaceae ACT-SP. Hn R G A
Mabberley (1997 p. 10) indicates Radix Christopherianae (Amer. Pharm.) to be a form of *Actaea spicata*.

Adenandra uniflora (L.) Willd., Enum. Pl. 256. 1809.
Rutaceae DIOSM.
Diosma uniflora L., Sp. Pl. 1: 198. 1753.
Diosma linearis Thunb., Prodr. Pl. Cap. 43. 1794.
Diosma "lincaris" (Comp. Rep.) appears to be a typographic error, the nearest combination is *Diosma linearis*.

Adhatoda vasica Nees, Pl. Asiat. Rar. 3: 103. 1832.
Acanthaceae JUST. Hs G
Justicia adhatoda L., Sp. Pl. 1: 15. 1753. Hn R

Adlumia fungosa (Aiton) Greene ex Britton, Sterns & Poggenb., Prelim. Cat. 3. 1888.
Papaveraceae ADLU. Hn R G

Fumaria fungosa Aiton, Hort. Kew. 3: 1. 1789.

Adonis vernalis L., Sp. Pl. 1: 547. 1753.
Ranunculaceae ADON. Hn R G A F

Adoxa moschatellina L., Sp. Pl. 1: 367. 1753.
Adoxaceae ADOX. Hn R

Aegle marmelos (L.) Corrêa, Trans. Linn. Soc. London 5: 223 1800.
Rutaceae AEGLE. Hn R
Crateva marmelos L., Sp. Pl. 1: 444. 1753.

Aegopodium podagraria L., Sp. Pl. 1: 265. 1753.
Apiaceae AEGO-P. Hn R

Aesculus carnea see *Aesculus glabra*

Aesculus glabra Willd., Enum. Pl. 405. 1809.
Hippocastanacea AESC-G. Hn R A
Aesculus rubicunda Lodd., Bot. Cab. 13: pl. 1242. 1827, incertae sedis. A
Aesculus carnea P. Watson, Dendrol. Brit. 2. t. 121. 1823 -1825, incertae sedis. A

Aesculus hippocastanum L., Sp. Pl. 1: 344. 1753.
Hippocastanacea AESC. Hn R G A F

Aesculus rubicunda see *Aesculus glabra*

Aethusa cynapium L., Sp. Pl. 1: 256. 1753.
Apiaceae AETH. Hn R G A F

Agaricus bulbosus see *Amanita phalloides*

Agaricus campanulatus see *Panaeolus papilionaceus*

Agaricus campestris L.: Fr., Sp. Pl. 2: 1173. 1753; Syst. Mycol. 1: 281. 1821.
Agaricaceae AGAR-CPS Hn R

Agaricus citrinus see *Amanita citrina*

Agaricus emeticus see *Russula emetica*

Agaricus muscarius see *Amanita muscaria*

Agaricus pantherinus see *Amanita pantherina*

Agaricus papilionaceus see *Panaeolus papilionaceus*

Agaricus phalloides see *Amanita phalloides*

Agaricus procerus see *Macrolepiota procera*

Agaricus semiglobatus see *Stropharia semiglobata*

Agaricus stercorarius see *Coprinus stercorarius*

Agathosma crenulata (L.) Pillans, J. S. African Bot. 16: 73. 1950.
Rutaceae. BAROS. R
Diosma crenulata L., Cent. Pl. 2, 11. 1756.

Diosma serratifolia Curtis, Bot. Mag. 13. t. 456. 1799.
Diosma crenata L., Syst. Nat. ed. 10, 2: 940. 1759. A
Barosma serratifolia (Curtis) Willd., Enum. Pl. 257. 1809.
Barosma crenulata Hook., Bot. Mag. 62. t. 3413. 1835. Hs A
Common homeopathic name: Buchu.

Agave americana L., Sp. Pl. 1: 323. 1753.
Agavaceae AGAV-A. Hn R A

Agave atrovirens see *Agave tequilana*

Agave tequilana F. A. C.Weber, Bull. Mus. Hist. Nat. (Paris) 8: 220, f. 1-2. 1902.
Agavaceae AGAV-T. Hn R A
Incorrect usage: *Agave atrovirens* sensu Amer. Pharm., not Karw.

Ageratina aromatica (L.) Spach, Hist. Nat. Vég. 10: 286. 1841.
Asteraceae EUP-A. R
Eupatorium aromaticum L., Sp. Pl. 2: 839. 1753. Hn
Incorrect usage: *Eupatorium urticifolium* (Hom. syn.) not Reichard.

Agnus castus see *Vitex agnus-castus*

Agraphis nutans see *Hyacinthoides non-scripta*

Agrimonia eupatoria L., Sp. Pl. 1: 448. 1753.
Rosaceae AGRI. Hn R

Agropyron repens (L.) P. Beauv., Ess. Agrostogr. 102, 146, 180, t. 20, f. 2. 1812.
Poaceae TRITIC. R G A F
Triticum repens L., Sp. Pl. 1: 86. 1753. Hn A
Elymus repens (L.) Gould, Madroño 9(4): 127. 1947. F

Agrostemma githago L., Sp. Pl. ed. 2, 1: 624. 1762.
Caryophyllaceae AGRO. Hn R A

Ailanthus altissima (Mill.) Swingle, J. Wash. Acad. Sci. 6: 495. 1916.
Simaroubaceae AIL. Hs G
Toxicodendron altissima Mill., Gard. Dict. ed. 8. "Toxicodendron" 10. 1768.
Ailanthus glandulosa Desf., Mém. Acad. Sci. (Paris) 1786: 265, t. 8. 1788. Hn R A

Ailanthus glandulosa see *Ailanthus altissima*

Alarconia helenioides see *Wyethia helenioides*

Alceae egyptiaceae see *Abelmoschus moschatus*

Aletris farinosa L., Sp. Pl. 1: 319. 1753.
Melanthiaceae ALET. Hn R G A F

Alfalfa see *Medicago sativa*

Allium cepa L., Sp. Pl. 1: 300. 1753.
Alliaceae ALL-C. Hn R G A F

Allium sativum L., Sp. Pl. 1: 296. 1753.
　　Alliaceae ALL-S. Hn R G A F

Alnus rubra see *Alnus serrulata*

Alnus serrulata (Aiton) Willd., Willd., Sp. Pl. 4(1): 336. 1805.
　　Betulaceae ALN. A
　　Betula serrulata Aiton, Hort. Kew. 1: 338. 1789.
　　Alnus rubra Desf. ex Spach, Ann. Sci. Nat. Bot. sér. 2, 15: 206.1841, not Bong. 1833. Hn R

Aloe ferox see *Aloe succotrina*

Aloe soccotrina see *Aloe succotrina*

Aloe socotrina see *Aloe succotrina*

Aloe succotrina Lam., Encycl. 1: 85. 1783.
　　Aloeaceae ALOE Hs
　　Aloe soccotrina Garsault, Fig. Pl. Méd. 1: t. 102. 1764.
　　Aloe soccotrina DC., Pl. Hist. Succ. 85, pl. 86. 1802.
　　Aloe "socotrina" (Comp. Rep. and Amer. Pharm.) is an orthographic variant. All three pharmacopoeias use different species and hybrids of Aloe. The French and the German pharmacopoeias use *Aloe ferox* Mill. The original homeopathic provings were of *Aloe socotrina*.

Alsidium helminthochorton (Tourr.) Kütz., Phycol. General. 435. 1843.
　　Rhodomelaceae HELM.
　　Fucus helminthochorton Tourr., Diss. Bot. J. Phys., Observ. Phys. 20: 183. 1782.
　　Alsidium "helmintochortos" (Comp. Rep.) is an orthographic variant. The combination "*Alsidium helminthochorton*" was made by Kütz., without any reference to the basionym, author, description or publication. Helmintochortos, the name used in homeopathy, is trivial.

Alsidium helmintochortos see *Alsidium helminthochorton*

Alsine media see *Stellaria media*

Alstonia constricta F.Muell., Fragm. 1: 57. 1858-1859.
　　Apocynaceae ALST-C. Hn R

Alstonia scholaris (L.) R. Br., Mem. Wern. Nat. Hist. Soc. 1: 76. 1809.
　　Apocynaceae ALST-S. Hn R A
　　Echites scholaris L., Mant. Pl. 1: 53. 1767. A

Alternanthera repens (L.) Kuntze, Revis. Gen. Pl. 2. 536. 1891.
　　Amaranthaceae PARO-I. A
　　Achyranthes repens L., Sp. Pl. 1: 205. 1753.
　　Paronychia illecebrum (Comp. Rep.) is an unknown combination. Tiangius pepetia (Hom. name and Amer. Pharm) is the vernacular name for *Alternanthera repens*.

Althaea officinalis L., Sp. Pl. 2: 686. 1753.
　　Malvaceae ALTH. Hn R A

Amanita citrina (Schaeff.: Fr) Gray, Nat. Arr. Brit. Pl. 1: 599. 1821.
Amanitaceae AGAR-CIT.
Agaricus citrinus Schaeff.: Fr., Fung. Bavar. Palat. Nasc. 1: 11. t. 20. 1762; Syst. Mycol. 1: 15. 1821. Hn R

Amanita muscaria (L.: Fr.) Hook., Fl. Scot. 19. 1821.
Amanitaceae AGAR. R A F
Agaricus muscarius L.: Fr., Sp. Pl. 2: 1172. 1753; Syst. Mycol. 1: 16. 1821. Hn A

Amanita pantherina (DC.: Fr) Krombh., Naturgetr. Abbild. Schwämme 4, pl. 29. 1836.
Amanitaceae AGAR-PA. R
Agaricus pantherinus DC.: Fr., Fl. Franç. 6: 52. 1815; Syst. Mycol. 1: 16. 1821. Hn

Amanita phalloides (Fr.: Fr.) Link, Handbuch 3: 272. 1833.
Amanitaceae AGAR-PH. R
Agaricus phalloides Fr.: Fr., Syst. Mycol. 1: 13. 1821. Hn
Agaricus bulbosus Bull., Hist Champ. France II. Première partie, pl. 577. 1809. Hs
Incorrect usage: *Amanita phalloides* sensu Germ. Pharm., not (Vaill. ex. Fr) Secretan.

Ambrina ambrosioides see *Chenopodium ambrosioides*

Ambroma augusta (L.) L. f., Suppl. Pl. 341. 1782.
Sterculiaceae ABROM-AUG. Hs
Theobroma augusta L., Syst. Nat. ed. 12, 3: 233. 1767.
Abroma augusta (L.) L. f., Suppl. Pl. 341. 1782. "Ambromal". Hn R

Ambrosia artemisiifolia L., Sp. Pl. 2: 988. 1753.
Asteraceae AMBRO.
Ambrosia elatior L., Sp. Pl. 2: 987-988. 1753. A
Ambrosia "artemisiefolia" (Comp. Rep.) is a typographic error.

Ambrosia artemisiefolia see *Ambrosia artemisiifolia*

Ammoniacum gummi see *Dorema ammoniacum*

Amorphophallus konjac K. Koch, Berliner Allg. Gartenzeitung 166. 1858.
Araceae AMOR-R.
Amorphophallus rivieri Durieu ex Carrière, Rev. Hort. 573. 1871. Hn R

Amorphophallus rivieri see *Amorphophallus konjac*

Ampelodesmos mauritanica (Poir.) T. Durand & Schinz, Consp. Fl. Afric. 5: 874. 1894.
Poaceae ARUND.
Arundo mauritanica Poir., Voy. Barbarie 2: 104. 1789. Hn
Ampelodesmos "mauritanicus" (Comp. Rep.) is an orthographic variant.

Ampelodesmos mauritanicus see *Ampelodesmos mauritanica*

Ampelopsis quinquefolia see *Parthenocissus quinquefolia*

Amphipterygium adstringens (Schltdl.) Standl., Contr. U. S. Natl. Herb. 23: 673. 1923.
Anacardiaceae RAJA-S. R
Hypopterygium adstringens Schltdl., Linnaea 17: 636. 1843.
Juliania adstringens Schltdl., Linnaea 17: 746. 1843.
"Juliana" adstringens (Amer. Pharm.) is an orthographic variant.
Rajania subsamarata (Hom. name and Amer. Pharm.) is a nom. nud.

Amygdalae dulcis see *Prunus dulcis*

Amygdalus amara see *Prunus dulcis*

Amygdalus communis see *Prunus dulcis*

Amygdalus dulcis see *Prunus dulcis*

Amygdalus persica see *Prunus persica*

Anacardium occidentale L., Sp. Pl. 1: 383. 1753.
Anacardiaceae ANAC-OC. Hn R

Anacardium officinarum see *Semecarpus anacardium*

Anacardium orientale see *Semecarpus anacardium*

Anagallis arvensis L., Sp. Pl. 1: 148. 1753.
Primulaceae ANAG. Hn R G A F
Anagallis phoenicea Scop., Fl. Carniol. ed. 2, 1: 139. 1772. A

Anagallis phoenicea see *Anagallis arvensis*

Anagyris foetida L., Sp. Pl. 1: 374. 1753.
Fabaceae ANAGY. Hn R

Anamirta cocculus (L.) Wight & Arn., Prodr. Fl. Ind. Orient. 446. 1834.
Menispermaceae COCC. R G A F
Menispermum cocculus L., Sp. Pl. 1: 340. 1753. A
Cocculus indicus Royle, Ill. Bot. Himal. Mts. 61. 1834, incertae sedis. Hn
Anamirta paniculata Colebr., Trans. Linn. Soc. London 13: 66. 1822. A F
Linnaeus (1749 p. 58) uses *Cocculus indicus* as the medicinal name for *Menispermum cocculus*, and is also used in commerce.

Anamirta paniculata see *Anamirta cocculus*

Anantherum muricatum see *Vetiveria zizanioides*

Anatherum muricatum see *Vetiveria zizanioides*

Andira araroba see *Vataireopsis araroba*

Andrographis paniculata (Burm. f.) Nees, Pl. Asiat. Rar. 3: 116. 1832.
Acanthaceae ANDROG-P Hn R
Justicia paniculata Burm. f., Fl. Indica 9. 1768.

Andromeda arborea see *Oxydendrum arboreum*

Andropogon muricatum see *Vetiveria zizanioides*

Andropogon muricatus see *Vetiveria zizanioides*

Andropogon squarrosus see *Vetiveria zizanioides*

Androsace lactea L., Sp. Pl. 1: 142. 1753.
Primulaceae ANDR. Hn R

Anemone flavescens see *Pulsatilla patens*

Anemone hepatica see *Hepatica nobilis*

Anemone nuttalliana see *Pulsatilla patens*

Anemone patens see *Pulsatilla patens*

Anemone pratensis see *Pulsatilla pratensis*

Anemone pulsatilla see *Pulsatilla pratensis*

Anemopsis californica Hook. & Arn., Bot. Beechey Voy. 390. 1841.
Saururaceae ANEMPS. Hn R

Angelica archangelica see *Angelica atropurpurea*

Angelica atropurpurea L., Sp. Pl. 1: 251. 1753.
Apiaceae ANGE. Hn R
Incorrect usage: *Archangelica officinalis* sensu Fren. Pharm., not Hoffm., and *Angelica archangelica* sensu Germ. Pharm., not L.

Angelica polymorpha var. sinensis see *Angelica sinensis*

Angelica sinensis (Oliv.) Diels, Bot. Jahrb. Syst. 29(3-4): 500. 1900.
Apiaceae ANGE-S.
Angelica polymorpha Max. var. *sinensis* Oliv., Icon Pl. 20(4): t. 1999. 1891.
"Angelicae" sinensis (Comp. Rep.) is an orthographic variant.

Angelicae sinensis see *Angelica sinensis*

Angophora costata subsp. **costata** (Gaertn.) Britten, Telopea 2(6): 756. 1986.
Myrtaceae ANGO.
Metrosideros costata Gaertn., Fruct. Sem. Pl. 1: 171. 1788.
Angophora lanceolata Cav., Icon. 4(1): 22, pl. 339. Sep-Dec 1797. Hn R

Angophora lanceolata see *Angophora costata* subsp. *costata*

Angostura cuspare see *Angostura trifoliata*

Angostura cusparia see *Angostura trifoliata*

Angostura trifoliata (Willd.) T. S. Elias, Taxon 19(4): 575. 1970.
Rutaceae ANG.
Bonplandia trifoliata Willd., Mém. Acad. Roy. Sci. Hist. (Berlin) 27. 1802. Hs A
Galipea officinalis J. Hancock, Trans. Med. Bot. Soc. London 1: 23, t. 11. 1829, nom. illeg. superfl. R G
Galipea cusparia A. St.-Hil. ex DC., Prodr. 1: 731. Jan 1824. Hs A F
Cusparia trifoliata (Willd.) Engl., Fl. Bras. 12(2): 113. 1874.

Angostura cuspare Roem. & Schult., Syst. Veg. 4: 188. 1819, nom. illeg.
Angostura "cusparia" (Amer. Pharm) is an orthographic variant. Angustura vera (Hom. name) is the name used in medicine.

Angostura vera see *Angostura trifoliata*

Anhalonium lewinii see *Lophophora williamsii* var. *lewinii*

Aniba coto (Rusby) Kosterm. ex J. F. Macbr., Publ. Field Mus. Nat. Hist., Bot. ser. 13(2): 863. 1938.
Lauraceae COTO
Nectandra coto Rusby, Bull. Torrey Bot. Club 49: 260. 1922. R
Common homeopathic name: Coto bark.

Anisum stellatum see *Illicium anisatum*

Annona triloba see *Asimina triloba*

Anthemis nobilis see *Chamaemelum nobile*

Anthemis vulgaris see *Matricaria recutita*

Anthoxanthum odoratum L., Sp. Pl. 1: 28. 1753.
Poaceae ANTHO. Hn R A

Antiaris toxicaria Lesch., Ann. Mus. Natl. Hist. Nat. 16: 478, pl. 22. 1810.
Moraceae UPA-A. R
Upas antiaris (Hom. name) is untraceable and appears to be a cannon of the common name upas tree with the generic epithet, *Antiaris*.

Antirrhinum linaria see *Linaria vulgaris*

Antirrhinum linarium see *Linaria vulgaris*

Apium crispum see *Petroselinum crispum*

Apium graveolens L., Sp. Pl. 1: 264. 1753.
Apiaceae AP-G. Hn R

Apium petroselinum see *Petroselinum crispum*

Apocynum androsaemifolium L., Sp. Pl. 1: 213. 1753. (corr. L., Syst. Nat., ed. 10, 2: 946. 1759).
Apocynaceae APOC-A. Hn R A

Apocynum cannabinum L., Sp. Pl. 1: 213. 1753.
Apocynaceae APOC. Hn R G A
Apocynum pubescens R. Br., Mem. Wern. Nat. Hist. Soc. 1: 68. 1809. A
Apocynum hypericifolium Aiton, Hort. Kew. 1: 304. 1789. A

Apocynum hypericifolium see *Apocynum cannabinum*

Apocynum pubescens see *Apocynum cannabinum*

Aquilegia vulgaris L., Sp. Pl. 1: 533. 1753.
Ranunculaceae AQUIL. Hn R G

Aragallus lamberti see *Oxytropis lambertii*

Aragallus lambertii see *Oxytropis lambertii*

Aralia hispida Vent., Descr. Pl. Nouv. t. 41. 1801.
Araliaceae ARAL-H. Hn R
For additional description see Michx., Fl. Bor.-Amer. ed. 1, 1: 185. 1803.

Aralia quinquefolia Decne. & Planch., Rev. Hort., ser. 4, 3: 105. 1854.
Araliaceae GINS. Hs A
Panax quinquefolium L., Sp. Pl. 2: 1058. 1753.
Incorrect usage: *Panax pseudoginseng* sensu Germ. Pharm., not Wall.
Linnaeus (1749 p. 39) uses Ginseng (Hom. name) as the medicinal name for *Panax quinquefolium*. *Panax "quinquefolius"* (Comp. Rep.) is an orthographic variant.

Aralia racemosa L., Sp. Pl. 1: 273. 1753.
Araliaceae ARAL. Hn R G A F

Arbutus andrachne L., Syst. Nat. ed. 10, 2: 1024. 1759.
Ericaceae ARBU. Hn R
Incorrect usage: *Arbutus unedo* (Hom. syn.) not L.

Arbutus menziesii Pursh, Fl. Amer. Sept. 1: 282. 1814.
Ericaceae ARB-M. Hn R

Arbutus unedo see *Arbutus andrachne*

Arbutus uva-ursi see *Arctostaphylos uva-ursi*

Archangelica officinalis see *Angelica atropurpurea*

Arctium lappa L., Sp. Pl. 2: 816. 1753.
Asteraceae LAPPA R A
Lappa major Gaertn., Fruct. Sem. Pl. 2(3): 379, pl. 162. 1791. A F
Lappa arctium Hill, Veg. Syst. 4, ed. 1, 28. 1762. Hn
Arctium majus (Gaertn.) Bernh., Syst. Verz. 154. 1800. F

Arctium majus see *Arctium lappa*

Arctostaphylos manzanita see *Arctostaphylos pungens*

Arctostaphylos pungens Kunth, Nov. Gen. Sp. 3: 278, t. 259. 1819.
Ericaceae MANZ.
Arctostaphylos manzanita Parry, Bull. Calif. Acad. Sci. 2: 491. 1887. R
Common homeopathic name: Manzanita.

Arctostaphylos uva-ursi (L.) Spreng., Syst. Veg. 2: 287. 1825.
Ericaceae UVA. R G A F
Arbutus uva-ursi L., Sp. Pl. 1: 395. 1753. A
Linnaeus (1749 p. 72) uses Uva-ursi (Hom. name) as the medicinal name for *Arbutus uva-ursi*.

Areca catechu L., Sp. Pl. 2: 1189. 1753.
Arecaceae AREC. Hn R

Argemone grandiflora see *Argemone mexicana*

Argemone mexicana L. Sp. Pl. 1: 508. 1753.
Papaveraceae ARGE. Hn R A
Argemone ochroleuca Sweet, Brit. Fl. Gard. ser. 1, 3: t. 242. 1827-1829. A
Argemone grandiflora Sweet, Brit. Fl. Gard. ser. 1, 3. t. 226. 1827-1829, incertae sedis. A

Argemone ochroleuca see *Argemone mexicana*

Arisaema atrorubens see *Arisaema triphyllum*

Arisaema dracontium (L.) Schott, Melet. Bot. 1. 17. 1832.
Araceae ARUM-D. R A
Arum dracontium L., Sp. Pl. 2: 964. 1753. Hn

Arisaema triphyllum (L.) Schott, Melet. Bot. 1: 17. 1832.
Araceae ARUM-T. R G A
Arum triphyllum L., Sp. Pl. 2: 965. 1753. Hn F
Incorrect usage: *Arisaema atrorubens* sensu Fren. Pharm., not (Aiton) Blume, and *Arum atrorubens* sensu Amer Pharm., not Aiton.

Aristolochia clematitis L., Sp. Pl. 2: 962. 1753.
Aristolochiaceae ARIST-CL. Hn R G A F

Aristolochia cymbifera Mart. & Zucc., Nov. Gen. Sp. Pl. 1: 76, t. 49. 1824.
Aristolochiaceae ARIST-M. R A
Aristolochia grandiflora Gomes, Mem. Math. Phis. Acad. Real Sci. Lisboa 3. 1812 in Mem. Corresp. 76. t. 3. (Date of publication could be 1814), not Arruda 1810, nor Sw. 1788. Hs
Mil-Homens is the vernacular name.

Aristolochia grandiflora see *Aristolochia cymbifera*

Aristolochia hastata see *Aristolochia serpentaria*

Aristolochia milhomens see *Aristolochia cymbifera*

Aristolochia officinalis see *Aristolochia serpentaria*

Aristolochia serpentaria var. hastata see *Aristolochia serpentaria*

Aristolochia serpentaria L., Sp. Pl. 2: 961. 1753.
Aristolochiaceae SERP. R A
Aristolochia serpentaria var. *hastata* (Nutt.) A. W. Wood, Class-book Bot. ed. s.n. (b): 602. 1861.
Aristolochia officinalis T. Nees, Pl. Medicin. pl. 144. 1828, incertae sedis. A
Aristolochia hastata Nutt., Gen. N. Amer. Pl. 2: 200. 1818. A
Linnaeus (1749 p. 147) uses Serpentaria virginiana (Hom. name) as the medicinal name for *Aristolochia serpentaria*.

Armoracia rusticana (Lam.) P. Gaertn., B. Mey. & Scherb., Oekon. Fl. Wetterau 2: 426. 1800.
Brassicaceae COCH. R A
Cochlearia rusticana Lam., Fl. Franç. 2: 471. 1778. A
Cochlearia armoracia L, Sp. Pl. 2: 648. 1753. Hn

Armoracia sativa Bernh., Syst. Verz. 189. 1800. Hs

Armoracia sativa see *Armoracia rusticana*

Arnica montana L., Sp. Pl. 2: 884. 1753.
Asteraceae ARN. Hn R G A F

Artemisia abrotanum L., Sp. Pl. 2: 845. 1753.
Asteraceae ABROT. R G A F
Artemisia paniculata Lam., Encycl. 1: 265. 1783. F
Linnaeus (1749 p. 135) uses Abrotanum (Hom. name) as the medicinal name for *Artemisia abrotanum*.

Artemisia absinthium L., Sp. Pl. 2: 848. 1753.
Asteraceae ABSIN. R Hs G A F
Linnaeus (1749 p. 136) uses Absinthium (Hom. name) as the medicinal name for *Artemisia absinthium*.

Artemisia cina see *Seriphidium maritimum*

Artemisia contra see *Seriphidium maritimum*

Artemisia heterophylla see *Artemisia vulgaris*

Artemisia heterophyllus see *Artemisia vulgaris*

Artemisia maritima see *Seriphidium maritimum*

Artemisia paniculata see *Artemisia abrotanum*

Artemisia vulgaris L., Sp. Pl. 2: 848. 1753.
Asteraceae ART-V. Hn R G A F
Artemisia heterophylla Nutt., Trans. Amer. Philos. Soc., n.s., 7: 400. 1840, incertae sedis.
Artemisia "heterophyllus" (Amer. Pharm.) is an orthographic variant.

Arum atrorubens see *Arisaema triphyllum*

Arum dracontium see *Arisaema dracontium*

Arum dracunculus see *Dracunculus vulgaris*

Arum italicum Mill., Gard. Dict. ed. 8. "Arum" 2. 1768.
Araceae ARUM-I. Hn R

Arum maculatum L., Sp. Pl. 2: 966. 1753.
Araceae ARUM-M. Hn R G A
Arum vulgare Lam., Fl. Franç. 3: 537. 1778. A

Arum seguine see *Dieffenbachia seguine*

Arum seguinum see *Dieffenbachia seguine*

Arum triphyllum see *Arisaema triphyllum*

Arum vulgare see *Arum maculatum*

Arundo mauritanica see *Ampelodesmos mauritanica*

Asafoetida see *Ferula narthex*

Asafoetida disgunensis see *Ferula narthex*

Asagraea officinalis see *Schoenocaulon officinale*

Asarum canadense L., Sp. Pl. 1: 442. 1753.
Aristolochiaceae ASAR-C. Hn R A

Asarum europaeum L., Sp. Pl. 1: 442. 1753.
Aristolochiaceae ASAR. Hn R G A

Asclepias amoena see *Asclepias incarnata*

Asclepias cornuti see *Asclepias syriaca*

Asclepias gigantea see *Calotropis gigantea*

Asclepias incarnata L., Sp. Pl. 1: 215. 1753.
Asclepiadaceae ASC-I. Hn R A
Asclepias amoena Brongn Ann. Sci. Nat. (Paris) ser. I, 24. 1831. not L. 1753.
{Publication not seen} A

Asclepias syriaca L., Sp. Pl. ed. 2, 1: 313. 1762.
Asclepiadaceae ASC-C. R A
Asclepias cornuti DC., Prodr. 8: 564. Mar 1844, incertae sedis. Hn A

Asclepias tuberosa L., Sp. Pl. 1: 217. 1753.
Asclepiadaceae ASC-T. Hn R A

Asimina triloba (L.) Dunal, Monogr. Anonac. 83. 1817.
Annonaceae ASIM. Hn R A
Annona triloba L., Sp. Pl. 1: 537. 1753. A
Uvaria triloba (L.) Torr. & A. Gray, Fl. N. Amer. 1(1): 45. 1838. Hs

Asparagus officinalis L., Sp. Pl. 1: 313. 1753.
Asparagaceae ASPAR. Hn R G A

Asperula odorata see *Galium odoratum*

Aspidium filix-mas see *Dryopteris filix-mas*

Aspidosperma quebracho see *Macaglia quebracho-blanco*

Aspidosperma quebracho-blanco see *Macaglia quebracho-blanco*

Asplenium scolopendrium L., Sp. Pl. 2: 1079. 1753.
Aspleniaceae SCOLO-V. R
Scolopendrium vulgare Sm., Mém. Acad. Roy. Sci. (Turin) 5(1791-1792): 421. 1793. Hn

Astragalus exscapus L., Mant. Pl. 2: 275. 1771.
Fabaceae ASTRA-E. Hn R

Astragalus lambertii see *Oxytropis lambertii*

Astragalus lambertii see *Oxytropis lambertii*

Astragalus menziesii see *Astragalus nuttallii*

Astragalus nuttallii (Torr. & A. Gray) J. T. Howell, Leafl. W. Bot. 5(6): 107. 1948.
Fabaceae ASTRA-ME.
Phaca nuttallii Torr. & A. Gray, Fl. N. Amer. 1(2): 343. 1838.
Astragalus menziesii A. Gray, Proc. Amer. Acad. Arts 6: 217. 1863, illegitimate substitute for Phaca densifolia Sm. Hn R

Athamanta oreoselinum see *Peucedanum oreoselinum*

Athamantha oreoselinum see *Peucedanum oreoselinum*

Atista indica see *Glycosmis pentaphylla*

Atriplex hortensis L., Sp. Pl. 2: 1053. 1753.
Chenopodiaceae ATRI. Hn R

Atropa belladonna L., Sp. Pl. 1: 181. 1753.
Solanaceae BELL. R Hs G A F
The terms bella and donna of the specific epithet have been united to conform to general usage rather than the hyphenated form, *bella-donna* recommended by the ICBN code 2000. Linnaeus (1749 p. 30) uses Belladonna (Hom. name) as the medicinal name for *Atropa belladonna*.

Aurantium maximum see *Citrus maxima*

Avena sativa L., Sp. Pl. 1: 79. 1753.
Poaceae AVEN. Hn R G A F

Azadirachta indica A. Juss., Mém. Mus. Hist. Nat. 19: 221, t. 13, 5. 1832.
Meliaceae AZA. Hn R
Melia azadirachta L., Sp. Pl. 1: 385. 1753. Hs

Balsamum peruvianum see *Myroxylon balsamum* var *pereirae*

Balsamum tolutanum see *Myroxylon balsamum*

Bambos arundinacea see *Bambusa arundinacea*

Bambusa arundinacea (Retz.) Willd., Willd., Sp. Pl. 2(1): 245. 1799.
Poaceae BAMB-A. Hn R
Bambos arundinacea Retz., Observ. Bot. 5: 24. 1789.

Banisteria caapi see *Banisteriopsis caapi*

Banisteriopsis caapi (Spruce ex Griseb.) C. V. Morton, J. Wash. Acad. Sci. 21: 486. 1931.
Malpighiaceae BANI-C. Hn R
Banisteria caapi Spruce ex Griseb., Fl. Brasil. 12(1): 43. 1858.

Bankesia abbyssinica see *Hagenia abyssinica*

Baptisia australis (L.) R. Br., Hortus Kew. 3: 6. 1811.
Fabaceae BAPT-C. R
Sophora australis L., Syst. Nat. ed. 12, 2: 287. 1767.

Baptisia confusa G. Don, Gen. Hist. 2: 113. 1832. Hn

Baptisia confusa see *Baptisia australis*

Baptisia tinctoria (L.) Vent., Dec. Gen. Nov. 9. 1808.
Fabaceae BAPT. Hn R A F
Sophora tinctoria L., Sp. Pl. 1: 373. 1753. A F
Podalyria tinctoria (L.) Willd., Willd., Sp. Pl. 2(2): 503. 1799.
Podalyria tinctoria (L.) Michx., Fl. Bor.-Amer. ed. 1, 1: 265. 1803, nom. illeg. Hs
Baptisia tinctoria (L.) R. Br., Hortus Kew. 3: 6. 1811. nom. illeg. superfl.

Barosma crenulata see *Agathosma crenulata*

Barosma serratifolia see *Agathosma crenulata*

Belladonna see *Atropa belladonna*

Bellis perennis L., Sp. Pl. 2: 886. 1753.
Asteraceae BELL-P. Hn R G A F

Benzoin see *Lindera benzoin*

Berberis aquifolium see *Mahonia aquifolium*

Berberis vulgaris L., Sp. Pl. 1: 330. 1753.
Berberidaceae BERB. Hn R G A F

Beta vulgaris L., Sp. Pl. 1: 222. 1753.
Chenopodiaceae BETA. Hn R

Betonica officinalis see *Stachys officinalis*

Betula serrulata see *Alnus serrulata*

Bignonia caroba see *Jacaranda caroba*

Bignonia sempervirens see *Gelsemium sempervirens*

Bixa orellana L., Sp. Pl. 1: 512. 1753.
Bixaceae BIX. Hn R

Blumea balsamifera (L.) DC., Prodr. 5: 447. Oct 1836.
Asteraceae BLUM-O. R
Conyza balsamifera L., Sp. Pl. ed. 2. 1208. 1763.
Blumea odorata (Hom. name) appears to be an unknown combination.

Blumea odorata see *Blumea balsamifera*

Boerhavia diffusa L., Sp. Pl. 1: 3. 1753.
Nyctaginaceae BOERH. Hn R

Boldea fragrans see *Peumus boldus*

Boldo fragrans see *Peumus boldus*

Boletus laricis see *Fomitopsis officinalis*

Boletus luridus Schaeff., Icon. Descr. Fung. t. 107. 1761.

Boletaceae BOL-LU. Hn R

Boletus pinicola see *Fomitopsis pinicola*

Boletus pinus see *Fomitopsis pinicola*

Boletus purgans see *Fomitopsis officinalis*

Boletus satanas Lenz, Nütz. Schädl. Schwämme 67. 1831. {Publication not seen}
Boletaceae BOL-S. Hn R

Bonplandia trifoliata see *Angostura trifoliata*

Borago officinalis L., Sp. Pl. 1: 137. 1753.
Boraginaceae BORAG. Hn R

Bovista gigantea see *Calvatia gigantea*

Bovista lycoperdon see *Calvatia gigantea*

Brachyglottis repanda J. R. Forst. & G. Forst., Char. Gen. Pl. ed. 1: 46. 1775.
Asteraceae BRACH. R
Millspaugh (1892, 1: 78-4) cites *Brachyglottis repens* Forsk, instead of *Brachyglottis repanda* Forst. This miscitation could account for the origin of the homeopathic name Brachyglottis repens.

Brachyglottis repens see *Brachyglottis repanda*

Brahea serrulata see *Serenoa repens*

Branca ursina see *Heracleum sphondylium*

Brassica alba (L.) Rabenh., Fl. Lusat. 1: 184. 1839.
Brassicaceae SIN-A. Hs A
Sinapis alba L., Sp. Pl. 2: 668. 1753. Hn R A

Brassica napus L., Sp. Pl. 2: 666. 1753.
Brassicaceae BRASS. Hn R

Brassica nigra (L.) W. Koch, Deutschl. Fl. ed. 3, 4: 713. 1833.
Brassicaceae SIN-N. Hs A
Sinapis nigra L., Sp. Pl. 2: 668. 1753. Hn R A

Brassica oleracea L., Sp. Pl. 2: 667. 1753.
Brassicaceae BRASS-O. Hn R G

Brauneria pallida see *Echinacea angustifolia*

Brayera anthelmintica see *Hagenia abyssinica*

Brosimum gaudichaudii Trécul, Ann. Sci. Nat., Bot. ser. 3, 8: 140. 1847.
Moraceae BROS-G. R

Brucea antidysenterica J. F. Mill., Icon. Anim. Pl. (1): t. 25. 1779 vel 1780.
Rutaceae BRUC. Hn R

Brugmansia arborea (L.) Lagerh., Bot. Jahrb. Syst. 20: 663. 1895.

Solanaceae DAT-A. R
Datura arborea L., Sp. Pl. 1: 179. 1753. Hn
Brugmansia candida Pers., Syn. Pl. 1: 216. 1805. A

Brugmansia candida see *Brugmansia arborea*

Brugmansia sanguinea (Ruiz & Pav.) D. Don, Brit. Fl. Gard. 3: t. 272. 1835.
Solanaceae DAT-S. R
Datura sanguinea Ruiz & Pav., Fl. Peruv. 2: 15. 1799. Hn

Brunfelsia hopeana see *Brunfelsia uniflora*

Brunfelsia uniflora (Pohl) D. Don, Edinburgh New Philos. J. 7: 85. 1829.
Solanaceae FRANC. R
Franciscea uniflora Pohl, Pl. Bras. Icon. Descr. 1: 2, t. 1. 1826. Hn
Brunfelsia hopeana Benth. in DC., Prodr. 10: 200. Apr 1846. Hs

Bryonia alba L., Sp. Pl. 2: 1012. 1753.
Cucurbitaceae BRY. Hn R A F
Incorrect usage: *Bryonia cretica* L. subsp. *dioica* sensu Germ. and Fren. Pharm not (Jacq.) Tutin.

Bryonia cretica subsp. dioica see *Bryonia alba*

Bryonia grandis see *Coccinia grandis*

Buchu see *Agathosma crenulata*

Bunias orientalis L., Sp. Pl. 2: 670. 1753.
Brassicaceae BUNI-O. Hn R

Buxus sempervirens L., Sp. Pl. 2: 983. 1753.
Buxaceae BUX. Hn R F

Cacao see *Theobroma cacao*

Cactus bonplandii see *Harrisia bonplandii*

Cactus ficus-indica see *Opuntia ficus-indica*

Cactus grandiflorus see *Selenicereus grandiflorus*

Cactus microdasys see *Opuntia microdasys*

Cactus opuntia see *Opuntia vulgaris*

Cactus serpentinus see *Cereus serpentinus*

Caesalpinia bonduc (L.) Roxb., Fl. Ind. ed. 1832. 2: 362. 1832.
Fabaceae CAESAL.
Guilandina bonduc L., Sp. Pl. 1: 381. 1753.
Caesalpinia bonducella (L.) Fleming, Asiat. Res. 11: 159. 1810. Hn R

Caesalpinia bonducella see *Caesalpinia bonduc*

Cainca see *Chiococca alba*

cajuput oil see *Melaleuca cajuputi*

Cajuputum see *Melaleuca cajuputi*

Caladium seguinum see *Dieffenbachia seguine*

Calea ternifolia Kunth, Nov. Gen. Sp. 4: 294. 1820.
Asteraceae CAEL.
Calea zacatechichi Schltdl., Linnaea 9: 589. 1834. Hn R A

Calea zacatechichi see *Calea ternifolia*

Calendula officinalis L., Sp. Pl. 2: 921. 1753.
Asteraceae CALEN. Hn R G A F

Calliandra houstoniana (Miller) Standl., Contr. U. S. Natl. Herb. 23(2): 386. 1922.
Fabaceae CALLI. Hn R
Mimosa houstoniana Mill., Gard. Dict. ed. 8. "Mimosa" 16. 1768.

Callicocca ipecacuanha see *Psychotria ipecacuanha*

Calonyction speciosum see *Ipomoea alba*

Calotropis gigantea (L.) R. Br., Hortus Kew. 2: 78. 1811.
Asclepiadaceae CALO. Hn R A
Asclepias gigantea L., Sp. Pl. 1: 214. 1753. A

Caltha arctica see *Caltha palustris*

Caltha palustris L., Sp. Pl. 1: 558. 1753.
Ranunculaceae CALTH. Hn R G A
Caltha arctica R. Br., J. Voy. n.-w. Passage, Bot. 265. 1824. A

Calvatia gigantea (Batsch: Pers.) Lloyd, Mycol. Not. 1: 166. 1904.
Lycoperdaceae BOV.
Lycoperdon gigantea Batsch.: Pers., Elench. Fung. 237. 1786; Synop. Meth. 140. 1801.
Lycoperdon bovista L., Sp. Pl. 2: 1183. 1753. Hs
Bovista gigantea Nees not Pers., Syst. f. 124. {Publication not seen}.
Bovista gigantea Bull, (Fren. Pharm.) and *Bovista lycoperdon* (Comp. Rep.) cannot be traced. *Lycoperdon bovista* L., is used in medicine and is most likely to be the species used in homeopathy. Linnaeus (1749 p. 176), also uses *Lycoperdon bovista* in his Materia Medica.

Calystegia spithamaea (L.) Pursh subsp. **stans** (Michx.) Brummitt, Ann. Missouri Bot. Gard. 52(2): 215. 1965.
Convolvulaceae CONVO-S.
Convolvulus stans Michx., Fl. Bor.-Amer. 1: 136. 1803. Hn
Incorrect usage: *Convolvulus spithamaeus* sensu Comp. Rep., not L. The homeopathic proving was of *Convolvulus stans*.

Camelia thea see *Camellia sinensis*

Camellia sinensis (L.) Kuntze, Trudy Imp. S.-Peterburgsk. Bot. Sada 10: 195 in obs. 1887.
Theaceae THEA. R

Thea sinensis L., Sp. Pl. 1: 515. 1753. Hn A
Camellia thea Link, Enum. Hort. Berol. Alt. 2: 73. 1822.
"Camelia" thea (Amer. Pharm.) is a typographic error.

Camellia thea see *Camellia sinensis*

Camphor officinarum see *Cinnamomum camphora*

Camphora see *Cinnamomum camphora*

Camphora officinarum see *Cinnamomum camphora*

Canchalagua see *Centaurium chironioides*

Candida albicans (C. P. Robin) Berkhout, Schimmelgesl. Monilia 41. 1923.
Aff. Metschnikowiaceae (Fungi) MONI.
Oidium albicans C. P. Robin, Hist. Nat. Vég. Paras. 488. 1853.
Monilia albicans (C. P. Robin) Zopf, Pilze 478. 1890. Hn R

Canna angustifolia see *Canna glauca*

Canna glauca L., Sp. Pl. 1: 1. 1753.
Cannaceae CANNA R A
Canna angustifolia L., Sp. Pl. 1: 1. 1753. Hn

Cannabis indica Lam., Encycl. 1: 695. 1785.
Cannabaceae CANN-I. Hn R A
Cannabis sativa subsp. *indica* (Lam.) E. Small & Cronquist, Taxon 25(4): 426. 1976. Hn R A
See Schultes et al. in Bot Mus. Leafl. Harvard Univ. 23: 337-367. 1974, for more information on the resolution of the accepted name.

Cannabis sativa subsp. indica see *Cannabis indica*

Cannabis sativa L., Sp. Pl. 2: 1027. 1753.
Cannabaceae CANN-S. Hn R A
For additional information see Bot. Mus. Leafl. Harvard Univ. 23: 333. 1974.

Capparis coriacea Burch. ex DC., Prodr. 1: 248. Jan 1824.
Capparaceae CAPP. Hn R

Capsella bursa-pastoris (L.) Medik., Pfl.-Gatt. 1: 85. 1792.
Brassicaceae THLASPI R G A F
Thlaspi bursa-pastoris L., Sp. Pl. 2: 647. 1753. Hn

Capsicum annuum L., Sp. Pl. 1: 188. 1753.
Solanaceae CAPS. Hn R G A F
Capsicum longum DC., Cat. Pl. Horti monsp. 86. 1813. A
Capsicum grossum Willd., Enum. Pl. 241. 1809. A

Capsicum grossum see *Capsicum annuum*

Capsicum longum see *Capsicum annuum*

Carduus benedictus see *Cnicus benedictus*

Carduus marianus see *Silybum marianum*

Carica papaya L., Sp. Pl. 2: 1036. 1753.
   Caricaceae PAP-V. R
   Papaya vulgaris A. DC., Encycl. 5: 2. 1804. Hn

Carissa schimperi see *Acokanthera schimperi*

Carpinus virginiana see *Ostrya virginiana*

Carpopogon pruriens see *Mucuna pruriens*

Carum petroselinum see *Petroselinum crispum*

Carya alba see *Carya tomentosa*

Carya tomentosa (Poir.) Nutt., Gen. N. Amer. Pl. 2: 221. 1818.
   Juglandaceae CARY.
   Juglans tomentosa Poir., Encycl. 4: 504. 1798.
   Carya alba (L.) K. Koch, see Howard and Staples in J. Arnold Arbor. 64: 527. 1983.
   Carya alba (Mill.) K. Koch, Dendrologie 1: 596. 1869, see Rehder J. Arnold Arbor. 26: 482. 1945, not Nutt. 1818. Hn R A

Cascara sagrada see *Rhamnus purshiana*

Cascarilla see *Croton eluteria*

Cassava see *Manihot esculenta*

Cassia acutifolia see *Senna alexandrina*

Cassia angustifolia see *Senna alexandrina*

Cassia fistula L., Sp. Pl. 1: 377. 1753.
   Fabaceae CASSI-F. Hn R

Cassia obovata see *Senna alexandrina*

Cassia senna see *Senna alexandrina*

Cassia sophera see *Senna sophora*

Castalia pudica see *Nymphaea odorata*

Castanea sativa Mill., Gard. Dict. ed. 8. "Castanea" 1. 1768.
   Fagaceae CAST-V. R A
   Castanea vesca Gaertn., Fruct. Sem. Pl. 1(1): 181. 1788.
   Castanea vesca Bunge, Mém. Sav. Étr. Acad. Petersb. 2: 136. 1835. Hn

Castanea vesca see *Castanea sativa*

Castela erecta Turpin subsp. **texana** (Torr. & A. Gray) Cronquist, Brittonia 5: 469. 1945.
   Simaroubaceae CHAP.
   Castela erecta Turpin, Ann. Mus. Natl. Hist. Nat. 7: 80, t. 5 B. 1806.
   Castela texana (Torr. & Gray) Rose, Contr. U.S. Natl. Herb. 12: 278. 1909.
   "*Castella*" *texana* (Amer. Pharm.) is a typographic error. Chaparro amargoso (Comp. Rep.) is an unknown combination and appears to be a cannon of the

vernacular names chaparro and amargosa.

Castela texana see *Castela erecta* subsp. *texana*

Castella texana see *Castela erecta* subsp. *texana*

Castiglionia lobata see *Jatropha curcas*

Catalpa bignonioides Walter, Fl. Carol. 64. 1788.
   Bignoniaceae CATAL. Hn R

Cataria nepeta see *Nepeta cataria*

Caulophyllum thalictroides (L.) Michx., Fl. Bor.-Amer. ed. 1, 1: 205. 1803.
   Berberidaceae CAUL. Hn R A F
   Leontice thalictroides L., Sp. Pl. 1: 312. 1753.

Ceanothus americanus L., Sp. Pl. 1: 195. 1753.
   Rhamnaceae CEAN. Hn R G A F

Ceanothus thyrsiflorus Eschsch., Mém. Acad. Imp. Sci. St. Pétersbourg Hist. Acad. 10: 285. 1826. "thyrsiflora".
   Rhamnaceae CEAN-TR. Hn R

Cecropia mexicana see *Cecropia obtusifolia*

Cecropia obtusifolia Bertol., Novi Comment. Acad. Sci. Inst. Bononiensis 4: 439. 1840.
   Cecropiaceae CECR. A
   Cecropia mexicana Hemsl., Biol. Cent.-Amer., Bot. 3: 151, t. 80. 1883. Hn R A

Cedron see *Simaba cedron*

Celtis occidentalis L., Sp. Pl. 2: 1044. 1753.
   Ulmaceae CELT. Hn R

Centaurea benedicta see *Cnicus benedictus*

Centaurea tagana Brot., Fl. Lusit. 1: 369. 1804.
   Asteraceae CENT. Hn R

Centaurium chironioides (A. Gray) Druce, Bot. Soc. Exch. Club Brit. Isles 1916: 613. 1917.
   Gentianaceae CANCH. R
   Erythraea chironioides A. Gray, Bot. California 1: 479. 1876. Hs
   The common name Canchalagua (Hom. name) refers to more than one species of *Centaurium*.

Centella asiatica (L.) Urb., Fl. Bras. 11(1): 287. 1879.
   Apiaceae HYDRC. G F
   Hydrocotyle asiatica L., Sp. Pl. 1: 234. 1753. Hn R A F
   Hydrocotyle nummularioides A. Rich., Monogr. Hydrocotyle 36. 1820.
   Hydrocotyle "nummulariodes" (Amer. Pharm) is a typographic error.

Cephaelis acuminata see *Psychotria ipecacuanha*

Cephaelis ipecacuanha see *Psychotria ipecacuanha*

Cephalandra indica see *Coccinia grandis*

Cephalanthus occidentalis L., Sp. Pl. 1: 95. 1753.
Rubiaceae CEPH. Hn R

Cerasus serotina see *Prunus virginiana*

Cerasus virginiana see *Prunus virginiana*

Cerbera manghas L., Sp. Pl. 1: 208. 1753.
Apocynaceae TANG.
Tanghinia venenifera Poir., Encycl. Suppl. 5: 283. 1817. Hn A
Cerbera venenifera (Poir.) Steud., Nomencl. Bot. ed. 2(1): 332. 1840.
Cerbera tanghin Hook., Bot. Mag. 57: t. 2968. 1830, nom. superfl.
Cerbera "tanghinia" (Comp. Rep.) is an orthographic variant.

Cerbera peruviana see *Thevetia peruviana*

Cerbera tanghin see *Cerbera manghas*

Cerbera tanghinia see *Cerbera manghas*

Cerbera thevetia see *Thevetia peruviana*

Cerbera venenifera see *Cerbera manghas*

Cereus bonplandii see *Harrisia bonplandii*

Cereus grandiflorus see *Selenicereus grandiflorus*

Cereus serpentinus (Lag. & Rodr.) DC., Prodr. 3: 467. Mar 1828.
Cactaceae CERE-S. Hn R
Cactus serpentinus Lag. & Rodr., Anales Ci. Nat. 4(12): 261. 1801.

Cessampelos pareira see *Chondrodendron tomentosum*

Cetraria islandica (L.) Ach., Methodus 293. 1803. sensu latiore.
Parmeliaceae CETR. Hn R G
Lichen islandicus L., Sp. Pl. 2: 1145. 1753.

Chamaecyparis lawsoniana (A. Murray bis) Parl., Ann. Mus. Imp. Fis. Firenze n.s., 1: 181. (preprint p. 29). 1864.
Cupressaceae CUPRE-L.
Cupressus lawsoniana A. Murray bis., Edinburgh New Philos. J. ser. 1, 292, pl. 9. 1855. Hn R

Chamaelirium luteum see *Helonias dioica*

Chamaemelum nobile (L.) All., Fl. Pedem. 1: 185. 1785.
Asteraceae ANTH. R G
Anthemis nobilis L., Sp. Pl. 2: 894. 1753. Hn A
Chamomilla nobilis Godr., Fl. Lorraine. ed. 1, 2: 19. 1843. A

Chamaesyce prostrata (Aiton) Small, Fl. s. e. U. S. ed. 1, 713, 1333. 1903.
Euphorbiaceae EUPH-PR.

Euphorbia prostrata Aiton, Hort. Kew. 2: 139. 1789. Hn R

Chamomilla see *Matricaria recutita*

Chamomilla nobilis see *Chamaemelum nobile*

Chamomilla recutita see *Matricaria recutita*

Chaparro amargoso see *Castela erecta* subsp. *texana*

Chaulmoogra see *Hydnocarpus kurzii*

Cheiranthus cheiri L., Sp. Pl. 2: 661. 1753.
 Brassicaceae CHEIR. Hn R G

Cheiranthus incanus see *Matthiola incana*

Chelidonium haematodes see *Chelidonium majus*

Chelidonium majus L., Sp. Pl. 1: 505. 1753.
 Papaveraceae CHEL. Hn R G A F
 Chelidonium haematodes Moench, Methodus 249. 1794. A

Chelone alba see *Chelone glabra*

Chelone glabra L., Sp. Pl. 2: 611. 1753.
 Scrophulariaceae CHELO. Hn R A
 Chelone alba Moench, Methodus 442. 1794. A

Chenopodium ambrosioides L., Sp. Pl. 1: 219. 1753.
 Chenopodiaceae CHEN-A. Hs G
 Chenopodium anthelminticum L., Sp. Pl. 1: 220. 1753. Hn R A
 Ambrina ambrosioides Spach, Hist. Nat. Vég. 5: 297. 1836. A

Chenopodium anthelminticum see *Chenopodium ambrosioides*

Chenopodium vulvaria L., Sp. Pl. 1: 220. 1753.
 Chenopodiaceae CHEN-V. Hn R

Chimaphila corymbosa see *Chimaphila umbellata*

Chimaphila maculata (L.) Pursh, Fl. Amer. Sept. 1: 300. 1814.
 Ericaceae CHIM-M. Hn R
 Pyrola maculata L., Sp. Pl. 1: 396. 1753.

Chimaphila umbellata (L.) W. Barton, Veg. Mater. Med. U.S. 1: 17. 1817.
 Ericaceae CHIM. Hn R G A F
 Pyrola umbellata L., Sp. Pl. 1: 396. 1753. F
 Pyrola corymbosa (Pursh) Bertol., Novi Comment. Acad. Sci. Inst. Bononiensis 6: 428. 1844, nom. illeg. A
 Chimaphila umbellata (L.) Nutt., Gen. N. Amer. Pl. 1: 274. 1818, nom.illeg. G
 Chimaphila corymbosa Pursh, Fl. Amer. Sept. 1: 300. 1814. A

China officinalis see *Cinchona officinalis*

Chiococca alba (L.) Hitchc., Annual Rep. Missouri Bot. Gard. 4: 94. 1893.

Rubiaceae CAHIN. R
Lonicera alba L., Sp. Pl. 1: 175. 1753.
Chiococca racemosa L., Syst. Nat. ed. 10, 2: 917. 1759. Hs A
Millspaugh (1892, 1: 76-2) indicates Cainca (Hom. name) to be *Chiococca alba*.

Chiococca racemosa see *Chiococca alba*

Chionanthus virginiana see *Chionanthus virginica*

Chionanthus virginica L., Sp. Pl. 1: 8. 1753.
Oleaceae CHION.
Chionanthus "virginicus" (Comp. Rep.) and *Chionanthus "virginiana"* (Fren. Pharm.) are orthographic variants.

Chionanthus virginicus see *Chionanthus virginica*

Chirata indica see *Swertia chirata*

Chondrodendron tomentosum Ruiz & Pav., Syst. Veg. Fl. Peruv. Chil. 261. 1798.
Menispermaceae PAREIR. R A F
Incorrect usage: *Cissampelos pareira* (Hom. syn.) not L. *"Cessampelos" pareira* (Hom. syn) is a typographic error. Common homeopathic name: Pareira brava.

Chrysanthemum leucanthemum see *Leucanthemum vulgare*

Chrysanthemum vulgare see *Tanacetum vulgare*

Chrysarobinum see *Vataireopsis araroba*

Cichorium intybus L., Sp. Pl. 2: 813. 1753.
Asteraceae CICH. Hn R G A

Cicuta maculata L., Sp. Pl. 1: 256. 1753.
Apiaceae CIC-M. Hn R A
Cicuta virosa var. *maculata* (L.) J. M. Coult. & Rose, Rev. N. Amer. Umbell. 130. 1888.

Cicuta major see *Conium maculatum*

Cicuta virosa var. maculata see *Cicuta maculata*

Cicuta virosa L., Sp. Pl. 1: 255. 1753.
Apiaceae CIC. Hn R A

Cimicifuga racemosa see *Actaea racemosa*

Cina see *Seriphidium maritimum*

Cinchona boliviana see *Cinchona officinalis*

Cinchona calisaya see *Cinchona officinalis*

Cinchona lancifolia see *Cinchona officinalis*

Cinchona officinalis L., Sp. Pl. 1: 172. 1753.

Rubiaceae CHIN. R A
Cinchona lancifolia Mutis, Papel Periodico de Santa Fe 111: 465. 1793.
{Publication not seen} A
Cinchona calisaya Wedd., Ann. Sci. Nat. Bot. sér. 3, 10: 6. 1848. Hs
Cinchona boliviana Wedd., Ann. Sci. Nat. Bot. sér. 3, 10: 7. 1848. R
Linnaeus (1749 p. 24) uses China (Hom. name) as the medicinal name for *Cinchona officinalis*. The synonym *Cinchona boliviana,* is cited as a separate remedy (CHIN-B) in the Complete Repertory. Other species of *Cinchona* namely, *Cinchona pubescens* Vahl, *Cinchona cordifolia* Mutis, and *Cinchona succirubra* Pav. ex Klotzsch, are also used by the major pharmacopoeias for the preparation of the homeopathic remedy, China.

Cinchona pubescens see *Cinchona officinalis*

Cinchona succirubra see *Cinchona officinalis*

Cineraria maritima see *Senecio bicolor* subsp. *cineraria*

Cinnamomum camphora (L.) J. Presl, Prir. rostlin 2: 47. 1823-25.
Lauraceae CAMPH. R G
Laurus camphora L., Sp. Pl. 1: 369. 1753. Hs
Camphora officinarum Nees, Pl. Asiat. Rar. 2: 72. 1831.
Linnaeus (1749 p. 65) uses Camphora (Hom. name) as the medicinal name for *Laurus camphora*. *"Camphor" officinarum* (Amer. Pharm.) is an orthographic variant.

Cinnamomum zeylanicum Breyne, Eph. Nat. Cur. Dec. 4: 139. 1789.
Lauraceae CINNAM. Hn R G A
Laurus cinnamomum L., Sp. Pl. 1: 369. 1753. A
Laurus cassia L., Sp. Pl. 1: 369. 1753, incertae sedis. A

Cissampelos pareira see *Chondrodendron tomentosum*

Cistus canadensis see *Helianthemum canadense*

Cistus helianthemum see *Helianthemum canadense*

Citrullus colocynthis (L.) Schrad., Linnaea 12: 414. 1838.
Cucurbitaceae COLOC. R A F
Cucumis colocynthis L., Sp. Pl. 2: 1011. 1753. A F
Colocynthis vulgaris Schrad., Index Seminum [Goettingen] 2. 1833. A
Linnaeus (1749 p. 157) uses Colocynthis (Hom. name) as the medicinal name for *Cucumis colocynthis*.

Citrullus lanatus (Thunb.) Matsum. & Nakai, Cat. Sem. Spor. Hort. Bot. Univ. Imp. Tokyo 30, no. 854. 1916.
Cucurbitaceae CUC-C. R
Momordica lanata Thunb., Prodr. Pl. Cap. 13. 1794.
Cucurbita citrullus L., Sp. Pl. 2: 1010. 1753. Hn

Citrus aurantium var decumana see *Citrus maxima*

Citrus decumana see *Citrus maxima*

Citrus limonum see *Citrus x limon*

Citrus maxima (Rumph. ex Burm.) Merr., Interpr. Herb. Amboin. 46, 296. 1917.
    Rutaceae CIT-D.
    Aurantium maximum Rumph. ex Burm., Herb. Amboin. Auct. Z 1, verso. 1755; Merr., Interpr. Herb. Amboin. 46, 296. 1917.
    Citrus decumana (L.) L., Syst. Nat. ed. 12, 508. 1767. Hn R
    Citrus aurantium var. *decumana* L., Sp. Pl. 2: 783. 1753.

Citrus sinensis see *Citrus x aurantium*

Citrus vulgaris see *Citrus x aurantium*

Citrus x aurantium L., Sp. Pl. 2: 783. 1753.
    Rutaceae CIT-V. R
    Citrus vulgaris Risso, Ann. Mus. Natl. Hist. Nat. 20: 190. 1813. Hn
    Citrus sinensis Pers., Syn. Pl. 2(1): 74. 1806. not Osbeck 1765. F

Citrus x limon (L.) Osbeck, Reise Ostindien 250. 1765, "limonia".
    Rutaceae CIT-L. R
    Citrus medica L. var. *limon* L., Sp. Pl. 2: 782. 1753.
    Citrus "limonum" (Hom. name) is an orthographic variant.

Claviceps purpurea (Fr.) Tul. & C. Tul., Ann. Sci. Nat. Bot. sér. 3, 20: 45. 1853.
    Clavicipitaceae SEC.
    Sphaeria purpurea Fr., Syst. Mycol. 2: 325. 1823.
    Secale cornutum Baldinger (Comp. Rep., and Hom. name) was frequently used until it was elucidated by Tulasne, who named the fungus *Claviceps*.

Clematis erecta see *Clematis recta*

Clematis recta L., Sp. Pl. 1: 544. 1753.
    Ranunculaceae CLEM. R G A
    Clematis erecta L., Syst. Nat. ed. 12, 377. 1767. Hn F

Clematis vitalba L., Sp. Pl. 1: 544. 1753.
    Ranunculaceae CLEM-VIT. Hn R F

Clerodendranthus stamineus (Benth.) Kudô, Mem. Fac. Sci. Taihoku Imp. Univ. 2: 117. 1929.
    Lamiaceae ORTHOS.
    Orthosiphon stamineus Benth., Pl. Asiat. Rar. 2: 15. 1830. Hn R

Clutia eluteria see *Croton eluteria*

Cnicus benedictus L., Sp. Pl. 2: 826. 1753.
    Asteraceae CARD-B. R Hs G A
    Centaurea benedicta (L.) L., Sp. Pl. ed. 2, 2: 1296. 1763. Hs A
    Carduus benedictus [Mattioli], is a pre-Linnaean name. Hn

Cnidoscolus urens (L.) Arthur, Torreya 21: 11. 1921.
    Euphorbiaceae JATR-U. R
    Jatropha urens L., Sp. Pl. 2: 1007. 1753. Hn

Coca see *Erythroxylum coca*

Coccinia grandis (L.) Voigt, Hort. Suburb. Calcutt. 59. 1845.
  Cucurbitaceae CEPHD.
  Bryonia grandis L., Mant. Pl. 1: 126. 1767.
  Cephalandra indica (Wight & Arn.) Naudin, Ann. Sci. Nat. Bot sér. 5, 5: 16. 1866, nom. illeg. fide Keraudren (1990). Hn R

Cocculus indicus see *Anamirta cocculus*

Cochlearia armoracia see *Armoracia rusticana*

Cochlearia officinalis L., Sp. Pl. 2: 647. 1753.
  Brassicaceae COCH-O. Hn R G

Cochlearia rusticana see *Armoracia rusticana*

Cocos maldivica see *Lodoicea maldivica*

Coffea arabica L., Sp. Pl. 1: 172. 1753.
  Rubiaceae COFF. R G F
  The remedy made from the unroasted coffee berries, is referred to as Coffea cruda.

Coffea cruda see *Coffea arabica*

Cola acuminata (P. Beauv.) Schott & Endl., Melet. Bot. 1: 33. 1832.
  Sterculiaceae KOLA. R
  Sterculia acuminata P. Beauv., Fl. Oware 1: 41, t. 24. 1805. Hs
  Common homeopathic name: Kola.

Colchicum autumnale L., Sp. Pl. 1: 341. 1753.
  Colchicaceae COLCH. Hn R G A F
  Colchicum commune Neck., Delic. Gallo-Belg. 1: 176. 1768. A

Colchicum commune see *Colchicum autumnale*

Coleus amboinicus see *Plectranthus amboinicus*

Coleus aromaticus see *Plectranthus amboinicus*

Collinsonia canadensis L., Sp. Pl. 1: 28. 1753.
  Lamiaceae COLL. Hn R G A F

Colocynthis see *Citrullus colocynthis*

Colocynthis vulgaris see *Citrullus colocynthis*

Comocladia dentata Jacq., Enum Syst. Pl. 12. 1760.
  Anacardiaceae COM. Hn R A

Conium maculatum L., Sp. Pl. 1: 243. 1753.
  Apiaceae CON. Hn R A F
  Coriandrum cicuta Crantz, Stirp. Austr. ed. 1, Fasc. 3: 100. 1767. A
  Cicuta major Lam., Fl. Franç. 3: 456. 1778. A

Convallaria majalis L., Sp. Pl. 1: 314. 1753.
  Convallariaceae CONV. Hn R G A F

Convolvulus arvensis L., Sp. Pl. 1: 153. 1753.
  Convolvulaceae CONVO-A. Hn R

Convolvulus duartinus see *Ipomoea alba*

Convolvulus jalapa see *Ipomoea purga*

Convolvulus pulcherrimus see *Ipomoea alba*

Convolvulus purga see *Ipomoea purga*

Convolvulus purpureus see *Ipomoea purpurea*

Convolvulus scammonia L., Sp. Pl. 1: 153. 1753.
  Convolvulaceae SCAM. R Hs
  Linnaeus (1749 p. 28) uses Scammonium (Hom. name) as the medicinal name for *Convolvulus scammonia*.

Convolvulus spithamaeus see *Calystegia spithamaea* subsp. *stans*

Convolvulus stans see *Calystegia spithamaea* subsp. *stans*

Convolvulus turpethum see *Operculina turpethum*

Conyza anthelmintica see *Vernonia anthelmintica*

Conyza balsamifera see *Blumea balsamifera*

Conyza canadensis (L.) Cronquist, Bull. Torrey Bot. Club 70: 632. 1943.
  Asteraceae ERIG. R G F
  Erigeron canadensis L., Sp. Pl. 2: 863. 1753. Hn F
  Erigeron pusillus Nutt., Gen. N. Amer. Pl. 2: 148. 1818. A
  Erigeron paniculatus Lam., Fl. Franç. 2: 141. 1778. A
  Erigeron "canadense" (Amer. Pharm.) is an orthographic variant.

Copaifera jacquinii see *Copaifera officinalis*

Copaifera officinalis (Jacq.) L., Sp. Pl. ed. 2, 1: 557. 1762.
  Fabaceae COP. R A
  Copaiva officinalis Jacq., Enum. Syst. Pl. 21. 1760. A
  Copaifera jacquinii Desf., Mém. Mus. Hist. Nat. 7: 376. 1821. A

Copaiva see *Copaifera officinalis*

Copaiva officinalis see *Copaifera officinalis*

Coprinus stercorarius [Bull.] Fr., Epicr. Syst. Mycol. 252: 1838.
  Coprinaceae AGAR-ST.
  Agaricus stercorarius Bull., Herb. France Pl. 542, f. 2. 1792. Hn R

Corallorhiza odontorhiza (Willd.) Poir., Dict. Sci. Nat. 10: 375. 1818.
  Orchidaceae CORH. Hn R
  Cymbidium odontorhiza Willd., Willd., Sp. Pl. 4(1): 110. 1805.

Coriandrum cicuta see *Conium maculatum*

Coriaria myrtifolia L., Sp. Pl. 2: 1037. 1753.
  Coriariaceae CORI-M. Hn R

Coriaria ruscifolia L., Sp. Pl. 2: 1037. 1753.
   Coriariaceae CORI-R. Hn R

Corn-smut see *Ustilago maydis*

Cornus alba see *Cornus sericea*

Cornus alternifolia L. f., Suppl. Pl. 125. 1782.
   Cornaceae CORN-A. Hn R

Cornus amomum see *Cornus sericea*

Cornus circinata L'Hér., Cornus 7. 1788.
   Cornaceae CORN. Hn
   Cornus rugosa Lam., Encycl. 2: 115. 1788. R A
   Cornus tomentulosa Michx., Fl. Bor.-Amer. ed. 1, 1: 91. 1803. A

Cornus florida L., Sp. Pl. 1: 117. 1753.
   Cornaceae CORN-F. Hn R A

Cornus lanuginosa see *Cornus sericea*

Cornus rugosa see *Cornus circinata*

Cornus sericea L., Mant. Pl. 2: 199. 1771.
   Cornaceae CORN-S. Hn R A
   Cornus lanuginosa Michx, Fl. Bor.-Amer. ed. 1, 1: 92. 1803. A
   Cornus amomum Mill., Gard. Dict. ed. 8. "Cornus" 5. 1768. A
   Cornus alba Pursh, Fl. Amer. Sept. 1: 109. 1814, not L. 1753. A

Cornus tomentulosa see *Cornus circinata*

Corydalis canadensis see *Dicentra canadensis*

Corydalis formosa see *Dicentra canadensis*

Corynocarpus laevigatus J. R. Forst. & G. Forst., Char. Gen. Pl. ed. 1: 16. 1775.
   Corynocarpaceae KARA. R
   Common homeopathic name: Karaka.

Corypha repens see *Serenoa repens*

Coto bark see *Aniba coto*

Cotyledon umbilicus Britten, Fl. Trop. Afr. 2: 398. 1871.
   Crassulaceae COT. Hn R A
   Incorrect usage: *Umbilicus pendulinus* sensu Amer. Pharm., not DC.

Coumarouna odorata see *Dipteryx odorata*

Crataegus laevigata (Poir.) DC., Prodr. 2: 630. Nov 1825.
   Rosaceae CRAT. Hs G F
   Mespilus laevigata Poir, Encycl. 4: 439. 1798.
   Crataegus oxyacantha L., Sp. Pl. 1: 477. 1753, nom. ambig. Hn R A F
   Crataegus oxyacantha auct. is the synonym of *Crataegus monogyna* Jacq.
   The different subspecies of *Crataegus oxyacantha* are synonyms of

Crataegus laevigata, Crataegus monogyna and other species. The Pharmacopoeias use a mixture of the different species.

Crataegus monogyna see *Crataegus laevigata*

Crataegus oxyacantha see *Crataegus laevigata*

Crateva marmelos see *Aegle marmelos*

Crocus sativus L., Sp. Pl. 1: 36. 1753.
Iridaceae CROC. Hn R G A F

Croton coccineus see *Mallotus philippensis*

Croton eluteria (L.) W. Wright, London Med. J. 8: 249. 1787; Reprinted in Mem. Late William Wright 207. 1828, not Benn. 1860.
Euphorbiaceae CASC. R A
Clutia eluteria L., Sp. Pl. 2: 1042. 1753.
Common homeopathic name: Cascarilla bark.

Croton philippensis see *Mallotus philippensis*

Croton tiglium L., Sp. Pl. 2: 1004. 1753.
Euphorbiaceae CROTO-T. Hn R G A F
Tiglium officinale Klotzsch, Nov. Actorum Acad. Caes. Leop.-Carol. Nat. Cur. 19(1): 418. 1843. Hs A F

Cubeba see *Piper cubeba*

Cucumis colocynthis see *Citrullus colocynthis*

Cucurbita citrullus see *Citrullus lanatus*

Cucurbita pepo L., Sp. Pl. 2: 1010. 1753.
Cucurbitaceae CUC-P. Hn R

Cundurango see *Marsdenia cundurango*

Cunila pulegioides see *Hedeoma pulegioides*

Cuphea viscosissima Jacq., Hort. Bot. Vindob. 2: 83, t. 177. 1772.
Lythraceae CUPH. Hn R

Cupressus lawsoniana see *Chamaecyparis lawsoniana*

Curcas purgans see *Jatropha curcas*

Curcuma longa L., Sp. Pl. 1: 2. 1753.
Zingiberaceae CURC. Hn R

Cusparia trifoliata see *Angostura trifoliata*

Cyclamen europaeum see *Cyclamen purpurascens*

Cyclamen officinalis see *Cyclamen purpurascens*

Cyclamen purpurascens Mill., Gard. Dict. ed. 8. "Cyclamen" 2. 1768.
Primulaceae CYCL. F
Cyclamen officinalis Wender. ex Steud., Nomencl. Bot. ed. 2(1): 458. 1840,

incertae sedis. A
Cyclamen europaeum auct. R G A
Incorrect usage: *Cyclamen vernum* sensu Amer. Pharm., not Sweet.

Cyclamen vernum see *Cyclamen purpurascens*

Cymbidium odontorhiza see *Corallorhiza odontorhiza*

Cymbopogon citratus (DC.) Stapf, Bull. Misc. Inform. Kew 322, 357. 1906.
Poaceae CYMBO-CI. R

Cynanchum indicum see *Tylophora indica*

Cynara cardunculus L., Sp. Pl. 2: 827. 1753.
Asteraceae CYNA.
Cynara scolymus L., Sp. Pl. 2: 827. 1753. Hn R A F

Cynara scolymus see *Cynara cardunculus*

Cynodon dactylon (L.) Pers., Syn. Pl. 1: 85. 1805.
Poaceae CYN-D. Hn R
Panicum dactylon L., Sp. Pl. 1: 58. 1753.

Cypripedium calceolus L. var. **pubescens** (Willd.) Correll, Bot. Mus. Leafl. 7: 14. 1938.
Orchidaceae CYPR. G F
Cypripedium pubescens Willd., Willd., Sp. Pl. 4(1): 143. 1805. Hn R A
Cypripedium luteum Aiton ex Raf., Med. Fl. 1: 142, t. 30. 1828. A

Cypripedium luteum see *Cypripedium calceolus* var. *pubescens*

Cypripedium pubescens see *Cypripedium calceolus* var. *pubescens*

Cytisus laburnum see *Laburnum anagyroides*

Cytisus scoparius (L.) Link, Enum. Hort. Berol. Alt. 2: 241. 1822.
Fabaceae SAROTH. R G A F
Spartium scoparium L., Sp. Pl. 2: 709. 1753.
Sarothamnus scoparius (L.) W. D. J. Koch, Syn. Fl. Germ. Helv. 152. 1835. Hn A

Dalbergia pinnata (Lour.) Prain, Ann. Roy. Bot. Gard. (Calcutta) 10(1): 48. 1904.
Fabaceae DER.
Derris pinnata Lour., Fl. Cochinch. 2: 432. 1790. Hn R
Dalbergia tamarindifolia Roxb., Fl. Ind. ed. 1832. 3: 233. 1832, prev. in Hort. Bengal. 53. 1814 as nom. nud.

Dalbergia tamarindifolia see *Dalbergia pinnata*

Damiana see *Turnera diffusa*

Daphne cannabina see *Daphne odora*

Daphne gnidium see *Daphne mezereum*

Daphne indica see *Daphne odora*

Daphne mezereum L., Sp. Pl. 1: 356. 1753.
 Thymelaceae MEZ. R G A F
 Incorrect usage: *Daphne gnidium* sensu Amer. Pharm., not L. Linnaeus (1749 p. 60) uses Mezereum as the medicinal name for *Daphne mezereum*.

Daphne odora Thunb., Nova Acta Regiae Soc. Sci. Upsal. 4: 39. 1783.
 Thymelaceae DAPH. R A
 Daphne indica Loisel., Herb. Amat. Fl. 2: t. 105. 1829.
 Daphne indica Hort. not L. 1753.
 Incorrect usage: *Daphne cannabina* sensu Amer. Pharm., not Wall., nor Hook. f (in part).

Datura arborea see *Brugmansia arborea*

Datura ferox L., Demonstr. Pl. 6. 1753.
 Solanaceae DAT-F. Hn R

Datura lurida see *Datura stramonium*

Datura metel L., Sp. Pl. 1: 179. 1753.
 Solanaceae DAT-M. Hn R

Datura sanguinea see *Brugmansia sanguinea*

Datura stramonium L., Sp. Pl. 1: 179. 1753.
 Solanaceae STRAM. R Hs G A F
 Stramonium foetidum Scop., Fl. Carniol. ed. 1, 157. 1760. A
 Datura lurida Salisb., Prodr. Stirp. Chap. Allerton 131. 1796. A
 Common homeopathic name: Stramonium.

Delphinium staphisagria L., Sp. Pl. 1: 531. 1753.
 Ranunculaceae STAPH.
 Linnaeus (1749 p. 94) uses Staphisagria (Hom. name) as the medicinal name for *Delphinium staphisagria*. *Delphinium "staphysagria"* (Comp. Rep.) is an orthographic variant.

Delphinium staphysagria see *Delphinium staphisagria*

Dendrobium punctatum see *Dipodium punctatum*

Dendrocnide sinuata (Blume) Chew, Gard. Bull. Straits Settlem. 21: 206. 1965.
 Urticaceae URT-C.
 Urtica sinuata Blume, Bijdr. Fl. Ned. Ind. 505. 1826.
 Urtica crenulata Roxb., Fl. Ind. ed. 1832. 3: 591. 1832, nom. illeg, not Sev. 1785. Hn
 Laportea crenulata Gaudich., Voy. Bonite, Bot. 498. 1846. R

Dens leonis see *Taraxacum officinale*

Derris pinnata see *Dalbergia pinnata*

Desmodium barbatum (L.) Benth., Pl. Jungh. 224. 1852.
 Fabaceae HEDY.
 Hedysarum barbatum L., Syst. Nat. ed. 10, 1170. 1759.

Hedysarum lagocephalum Link, Enum. Hort. Berol. Alt. 2: 248. 1822.
Hedysarum desmodium (Amer. Pharm.,and Hom. name) is an unknown name and appears to be a combination of two generic names. Millspaugh (1892, 1: 46-2) cites that *Hedysarum Ildefonsianum* Mure (Comp. Rep. and Amer. Pharm.) could be *Hedysarum lagocephalum* Link.

Desmodium gangeticum (L.) DC., Prodr. 2: 327. Nov 1825.
Fabaceae DESM-G. Hn R
Hedysarum gangeticum L., Sp. Pl. 2: 746. 1753.

Dicentra canadensis (Goldie) Walp., Repert. Bot. Syst. 1: 118. 1842.
Papaveraceae CORY. R
Corydalis canadensis Goldie, Edinburgh New Philos. J. 6: 329. 1822.
Corydalis formosa (Haw.) Pursh, Fl. Amer. Sept. 2: 462. 1814, incertae sedis. Hn

Dictamnus albus L., Sp. Pl. 1: 383. 1753.
Rutaceae DICT. A
Dictamnus fraxinella Pers., Syn. Pl. 1: 464. 1805. Hn R A

Dictamnus fraxinella see *Dictamnus albus*

Dieffenbachia seguine (Jacq.) Schott, Wiener Z. Kunst 803. 1829, {Publication not seen} see Dan H. Nicolson in Taxon 31: 550. 1982.
Araceae CALAD. R F
Arum seguine Jacq., Enum. Syst. Pl. 31. 1760.
Dieffenbachia seguine (Vent.) Schott, Melet. Bot. 1: 20. 1832.
Caladium seguinum Vent., Descr. Pl. Nouv. t. 30. 1801. Hn
Arum "seguinum" (Fren. Pharm., and Hom. syn.) is an orthographic variant of *Arum seguine*.

Digitalis purpurea L., Sp. Pl. 2: 621. 1753.
Scrophulariaceae DIG. Hn R G A F
Digitalis tomentosa Salisb., Prodr. Stirp. Chap. Allerton 100. 1796, incertae sedis. A

Digitalis tomentosa see *Digitalis purpurea*

Dilatris caroliniana see *Lachnanthes caroliniana*

Dioscorea paniculata see *Dioscorea villosa*

Dioscorea villosa L., Sp. Pl. 2: 1033. 1753.
Dioscoreaceae DIOS. Hn R G A F
Dioscorea paniculata Michx., Fl. Bor.-Amer. ed. 1, 2: 239. 1803. A

Diosma crenata see *Agathosma crenulata*

Diosma crenulata see *Agathosma crenulata*

Diosma lincaris see *Adenandra uniflora*

Diosma linearis see *Adenandra uniflora*

Diosma serratifolia see *Agathosma crenulata*

Diosma uniflora see *Adenandra uniflora*

Dipodium hamiltonianum see *Dipodium punctatum*

Dipodium punctatum (Sm.) R. Br., Prodr. ed. 1, 331. 1810.
Orchidaceae DIP. Hn
Dendrobium punctatum Sm., Exot. Bot. 1: 21, t. 12. 1804.
Dipodium punctatum var. *hamiltonianum* (Bailey) F. M. Bailey, Syn. Queensl. Fl. 517. 1883.
Dipodium hamiltonianum F. M. Bailey, Proc. Linn. Soc. New South Wales 6: 140. 1881. R

Dipteryx odorata (Aubl.) Willd., Willd., Sp. Pl. 3(2): 910. 1802.
Fabaceae TONG. R Hs
Coumarouna odorata Aubl., Hist. Pl. Guiane 2: 740, t. 296. 1775.
Millspaugh (1892, 1: 46-2) indicates Tongo (Hom. name) to be the Tonka bean (*Dipteryx odorata*).

Dirca palustris L., Sp. Pl. 1: 358. 1753.
Thymelaceae DIRC. Hn R A

Dolichos pruriens see *Mucuna pruriens*

Dolichos urens see *Mucuna urens*

Dorema ammoniacum D. Don, Trans. Linn. Soc. London 16: 602. 1833.
Apiaceae AMMC. R A
Dorema ammoniacum is the principle source of Ammoniacum gummi (Hom. name).

Dracontium foetidum see *Symplocarpus foetidus*

Dracunculus vulgaris Schott, Melet. Bot. 1: 17. 1832.
Araceae ARUM-DRU R
Arum dracunculus L., Sp. Pl. ed. 2, 2: 964. 1763. Hn

Drimia maritima (L.) Stearn, Ann. Mus. Goulandris 4: 204. 1978.
Hyacinthaceae SQUIL.
Scilla maritima L., Sp. Pl. 1: 308. 1753. Hs A
Urginea maritima (L.) Baker, J. Linn. Soc., Bot. 13: 221. 1873. R A
Common homeopathic name: Squill. *Urginea maritima* var. *alba* and *Scilla alba* are nomina nuda.

Drosera anglica see *Drosera rotundifolia*

Drosera intermedia see *Drosera rotundifolia*

Drosera rotundifolia L., Sp. Pl. 1: 281. 1753.
Droseraceae DROS. Hn R G A F
Rorella rotundifolia All., Fl. Pedem. 2: 88. 1785. A
The French and German pharamacopoeias also use *Drosera. intermedia* Hayne and *Drosera anglica* Huds.

Dryopteris filix-mas (L.) Schott, Gen. Fil. Fasc. 2, pl. 9. 1834.
Dryopteridaceae FIL. R G A

Polypodium filix-mas L., Sp. Pl. 2: 1090. 1753.
Aspidium filix-mas (L.) Sw., J. Bot. (Schrader) 1800(2): 38. 1801.
According to Stafleu, (1967 TL1), Genera Filicum is 20 lithographs in 4 fascicles. Each fascicle consists of 5 lithographs and 5 sheets of text. *Polystichum* including *Dryopteris* is cited as fascicle 2 pl. 9,but appears on pl. 17 of the BM copy. Filix-mas (Hom. name) is the name used in medicine.

Dulcamara see *Solanum dulcamara*

Ecballium elaterium (L.) A. Rich., Dict. Class. Hist. Nat. 6: 19. 1824.
Cucurbitaceae ELAT. R A
Momordica elaterium L., Sp. Pl. 2: 1010. 1753. Hs A
Linnaeus (1749 p. 157) uses Elaterium (Hom. name) as the medicinal name of *Momordica elaterium*.

Echinacea angustifolia DC., Prodr. 5: 554. Oct 1836.
Asteraceae ECHI. Hn R A F
Brauneria pallida (Nutt.) Britton, Mem. Torrey Bot. Club 5(22): 333. 1894. A
Rudbeckia pallida Nutt., J. Acad. Nat. Sci. Philadelphia 7: 77. 1834. A
Incorrect usage: *Rudbeckia angustifolia* sensu Fren. Pharm., not L.

Echinacea purpurea (L.) Moench, Methodus 591. 1794.
Asteraceae ECHI-P. Hn R G
Rudbeckia purpurea L., Sp. Pl. 2: 907. 1753.

Echites antidysenterica see *Holarrhena pubescens*

Echites pubescens see *Holarrhena pubescens*

Echites scholaris see *Alstonia scholaris*

Echites suberecta Andrews, Bot. Repos. 3: t. 187. 1801.
Apocynaceae ECHIT. Hn R

Eichhornia crassipes (Mart.) Solms, Monogr. Phan. 4: 527. 1883.
Pontederiaceae EICH-C. Hn R G
Pontederia crassipes Mart., Nov. Gen. Sp. Pl. 1: 9, pl. 4. 1823.

Elaeis guineensis Jacq., Select. Stirp. Amer. Hist. 280, pl. 172. 1763.
Arecaceae ELAE. Hn R

Elaterium see Ecballium elaterium

Elymus repens see *Agropyron repens*

Embelia ribes Burm. f., Fl. Indica 62, t. 23. 1768.
Myrsinaceae EMB. Hn R

Ephedra distachya L., Sp. Pl. 2: 1040. 1753.
Ephedraceae EPHE. Hn R G
Ephedra vulgaris Rich., Comm. Bot. Conif. Cycad. 26. 1826. Hs

Ephedra vulgaris see *Ephedra distachya*

Epifagus virginiana (L.) W. P. C. Barton, Comp. Fl. Philadelph. 50. 1818.

Scrophulariaceae EPIP.
Orobanche virginiana L., Sp. Pl. 2: 633. 1753. A
"Epiphegus" virginiana (Com. Rep.) is a typographic error.

Epigaea repens L., Sp. Pl. 1: 395. 1753.
Ericaceae EPIG. Hn R A

Epilobium angustifolium L., Sp. Pl. 1: 347. 1753.
Onagraceae EPIL-A. Hn R

Epilobium lineare see *Epilobium palustre*

Epilobium palustre L., Sp. Pl. 1: 348. 1753.
Onagraceae EPIL. Hn R
Epilobium lineare Muhl., Cat. Pl. Amer. Sept. ed. 1, 39. 1813, incertae sedis.
Hs

Epiphegus virginiana see *Epifagus virginiana*

Equisetum arvense L., Sp. Pl. 2: 1061. 1753.
Equisetaceae EQUIS-A. Hn R F

Equisetum hyemale L., Sp. Pl. 2: 1062. 1753.
Equisetaceae EQUIS. Hn R A F

Eranthis hyemalis (L.) Salisb., Trans. Linn. Soc. London 8: 304. 1807.
Ranunculaceae ERAN. Hn R
Helleborus hyemalis L., Sp. Pl. 1: 557. 1753.

Erechtites hieracifolia (L.) Raf. ex DC., Prodr. 6: 294. Jan 1838.
Asteraceae ERECH. Hn R A
Senecio hieraciifolius L., Sp. Pl. 2: 866. 1753.
Senecio "hieracifolius" (Amer. Pharm., and Hom. syn.) is a typographic error.

Erigeron canadense see *Conyza canadensis*

Erigeron canadensis see *Conyza canadensis*

Erigeron paniculatus see *Conyza canadensis*

Erigeron pusillus see *Conyza canadensis*

Eriodictyon californicum (Hook. & Arn.) Torr. Rep. U.S. Mex. Bound., Bot. 148. 1859.
Hydrophyllaceae ERIO. Hn R G A
Wigandia californica Hook & Arn., Bot. Beechey Voy 364, t. 88. 1839.

Erodium cicutarium (L.) L'Hér. ex Aiton, Hort. Kew. 2: 414. 1789.
Geraniaceae EROD. Hn R
Geranium cicutarium L., Sp. Pl. 2: 680. 1753.

Eryngium aquaticum L., Sp. Pl. 1: 232. 1753. not Hook. & Arn., 1841.
Apiaceae ERY-A. Hn R A
Incorrect usage: *Eryngium petiolatum* sensu Amer. Pharm., not Hook., and *Eryngium virginianum* sensu Amer. Pharm not Lam.

Eryngium maritimum L., Sp. Pl. 1: 233. 1753.
Apiaceae ERY-M. Hn R A

Eryngium petiolatum see *Eryngium aquaticum*

Eryngium virginianum see *Eryngium aquaticum*

Erythraea chironioides see *Centaurium chironioides*

Erythrina piscipula see *Piscidia piscipula*

Erythrophlaeum judiciale see *Erythrophleum suaveolens*

Erythrophleum guineense see *Erythrophleum suaveolens*

Erythrophleum judiciale see *Erythrophleum suaveolens*

Erythrophleum suaveolens (Guillem. & Perr.) Brenan, Taxon 9: 194. 1960.
Fabaceae ERYT-J.
Fillaea suaveolens Guillem. & Perr.Fl. Seneg. Tent. 1: 242, t. 55. 1832.
Erythrophleum judiciale Procter, Am. J. Pharm. 18: 195. 1852, incertae sedis.
{Publication not seen} A Hn
Erythrophleum guineense G. Don, Gen. Hist. 2: 424. 1832. R A
"Erythrophlaeum" judiciale (Hom. name) is an orthographic variant.

Erythroxylum coca Lam., Encycl. 2: 393. 1786.
Erythroxylaceae COCA R A
Common homeopathic name: Coca.

Eschscholzia californica Cham., Horae Phys. Berol. 73, t. 15. 1820.
Papaveraceae ESCH. Hn R F

Espeletia grandiflora Kunth, Pl. Aequinoct. 2: 11, t. 70. 1809.
Asteraceae ESP-G. Hn R

Eucalyptus globulus Labill., Voy. Rech. Pérouse 1: 153, t. 13. 1799.
Myrtaceae EUCAL. Hn R G A

Eucalyptus rostata see *Eucalyptus rostrata*

Eucalyptus rostrata Cav., Icon. 4(1): 23, pl. 342. Sep-Dec 1797 not Schltdl. 1847.
Myrtaceae EUCAL-R.
Eucalyptus "rostata" (Comp. Rep.) is a typographic error.

Eucalyptus tereticornis Sm., Spec. Bot. New Holland 4: 41. Jan. 1795.
Myrtaceae EUCAL-T. Hn R

Eugenia chequen see *Luma chequen*

Eugenia jambolana see *Syzygium cumini*

Eugenia jambolanum see *Syzygium cumini*

Eugenia jambos see *Syzygium jambos*

Euonymus atropurpureus Jacq., Hort. Bot. Vindob. 2: 55. 1772.

Celastraceae EUON-A. Hn R A

Euonymus europaea L., Sp. Pl. 1: 197. 1753.
Celastraceae EUON. Hn R G A

Eupatorium aromaticum see *Ageratina aromatica*

Eupatorium connatum see *Eupatorium perfoliatum*

Eupatorium maculatum see *Eupatorium purpureum*

Eupatorium perfoliatum L., Sp. Pl. 2: 838. 1753.
Asteraceae EUP-PER. Hn R G A F
Eupatorium salviaefolium Sims, Bot. Mag. 45. t. 2010. 1818. A
Eupatorium connatum Michx., Fl. Bor.-Amer. ed. 1, 2: 99. 1803. A

Eupatorium purpureum L., Sp. Pl. 2: 838. 1753.
Asteraceae EUP-PUR. Hn R G A
Eupatorium verticillatum Lam, Encycl. 2: 405. 1788. A
Eupatorium trifoliatum L., Sp. Pl. 2: 837. 1753. A
Eupatorium maculatum L., Cent. Pl. 1, 27. 1755; Amoen. Acad. 4(62): 288. 1759. A

Eupatorium salviaefolium see *Eupatorium perfoliatum*

Eupatorium trifoliatum see *Eupatorium purpureum*

Eupatorium urticifolium see *Ageratina aromatica*

Eupatorium verticillatum see *Eupatorium purpureum*

Euphorbia amygdaloides L., Sp. Pl. 1: 463. 1753.
Euphorbiaceae EUPH-A. Hn R

Euphorbia corollata L., Sp. Pl. 1: 459. 1753.
Euphorbiaceae EUPH-C. Hn R A

Euphorbia cyparissias L., Sp. Pl. 1: 461. 1753.
Euphorbiaceae EUPH-CY. Hn R G

Euphorbia heterodoxa Müll. Arg., Fl. Bras. 11(2): 701. 1874.
Euphorbiaceae EUPH-HE. Hn R

Euphorbia hirta L., Sp. Pl. 1: 454. 1753.
Euphorbiaceae EUPH-PI.
Euphorbia pilulifera L., Sp. Pl. 1: 454. 1753. Hn R

Euphorbia hypericifolia L., Sp. Pl. 1: 454. 1753.
Euphorbiaceae EUPH-HY. Hn R A

Euphorbia ipecacuanha see *Euphorbia ipecacuanhae*

Euphorbia ipecacuanhae L., Sp. Pl. 1: 455. 1753.
Euphorbiaceae EUPH-IP.
Euphorbia "ipecacuanha" (Comp. Rep.) is a typographic error.

Euphorbia lathyrus L., Sp. Pl. 1: 457. 1753.

Euphorbiaceae EUPH-L. Hn R

Euphorbia officinarum L., Sp. Pl. 1: 451. 1753.
Euphorbiaceae EUPH. Hs A
Incorrect usage: *Euphorbia resinifera* sensu Comp. Rep., Germ. and Amer Pharm., not O. Berg,. Common homeopathic name: Euphorbium.

Euphorbia peplus L., Sp. Pl. 1: 456. 1753.
Euphorbiaceae EUPH-PE. Hn R

Euphorbia pilulifera see *Euphorbia hirta*

Euphorbia polycarpa Benth., Bot. Voy. Sulphur 3: 50. 1844.
Euphorbiaceae EUPH-PO. Hn R

Euphorbia prostrata see *Chamaesyce prostrata*

Euphorbia resinifera see *Euphorbia officinarum*

Euphorbium see *Euphorbia officinarum*

Euphrasia latifolia see *Euphrasia officinalis*

Euphrasia officinalis L., Sp. Pl. 2: 604. 1753.
Scrophulariaceae EUPHR. Hn R G A F
Euphrasia latifolia Pursh, Fl. Amer. Sept. 2: 430. 1814. A

Euryangium sumbul see *Ferula sumbul*

Exogonium purga see *Ipomoea purga*

Eysenhardtia polystachia see *Eysenhardtia polystachya*

Eysenhardtia polystachya (Ortega) Sarg., Silva 3: 29. 1892.
Fabaceae EYS. Hn R
Viborquia polystachya Ortega, Nov. Pl. Descr. Dec. 66. 1798.
Eysenhardtia "polystachia" (Comp. Rep.) is a typographic error.

Fabiana imbricata Ruiz & Pav., Fl. Peruv. 2: 12, t. 122. 1799.
Solanaceae FAB. Hn R

Fagopyrum esculentum Moench, Methodus 290. 1794.
Polygonaceae FAGO. Hn R G A F
Polygonum fagopyrum L., Sp. Pl. 1: 364. 1753. Hs A F

Fagus sylvatica L., Sp. Pl. 2: 998. 1753.
Fagaceae FAGU. Hn R

Ferula asafoetida see *Ferula narthex*

Ferula communis L., Sp. Pl. 1: 246. 1753.
Apiaceae FERUL. R
Ferula neapolitana Ten., Fl. Napol. 3: 340, t. 182. 1824-1829. Hs
Ferula glauca L., Sp. Pl. 1: 247. 1753. Hn

Ferula glauca see *Ferula communis*

Ferula narthex Boiss., Fl. Orient. 2: 994. 1872.

Apiaceae ASAF. R A
Narthex asafoetida Falc. ex Lindl., Athenaeum (London) 996, 1222. 1846.
D.J. Mabberley in Taxon 31: 71. 1982. Hs
Linnaeus (1749 p. 40) uses Asafoetida (Hom. name) as the medicinal name.
Asafoetida resins are obtained from a variety of sources including *Ferula assa-foetida* auct., and *Asafoetida disgunensis* Kaempf. (Amer. Pharm.)

Ferula neapolitana see *Ferula communis*

Ferula sumbul (Kauffm.) Hook. f., Bot. Mag. 101: t. 6196. 1875.
Apiaceae SUMB. R Hs A
Euryangium sumbul Kauffm., Nouv. Mém. Soc. Imp. Naturalistes Moscou 13: 258. 1871.
Ferula sumbul is also referred to as the Sumbul plant (Hom. name) in Curtis Bot. Mag. 1875.

Ficus benghalensis L., Sp. Pl. 2: 1059. 1753.
Moraceae FIC-I.
Ficus indica L. not auct, Sp. Pl. 2: 1060. 1753. Hn R

Ficus carica see *Ficus religiosa*

Ficus Indica see *Ficus benghalensis*

Ficus religiosa L., Sp. Pl. 2: 1059. 1753.
Moraceae FIC. Hn R
Incorrect usage: *Ficus carica* sensu Fren. Pharm., not L.

Ficus tsjakela Burm. f., Fl. Indica 227. 1768.
Moraceae FIC-V. R
Ficus venosa Dryand., Hort. Kew. 3: 451. 1789. Hn

Ficus venosa see *Ficus tsjakela*

Filipendula ulmaria (L.) Maxim., Trudy Imp. S.-Peterburgsk. Bot. Sada 6(1): 251. 1879.
Rosaceae SPIRAE. R G F
Spiraea ulmaria L., Sp. Pl. 1: 490. 1753. Hn

Filix-mas see *Dryopteris filix-mas*

Fillaea suaveolens see *Erythrophleum suaveolens*

Flor de piedra see *Lophophytum leandrii*

→ **Fomitopsis officinalis** (Vill.: Fr.) Bondartsev & Singer, Ann. Mycol. 39: 55. 1941.
Coriolaceae BOL.
Polyporus officinalis Vill.: Fr., Syst. Mycol. I: 365. 1821. Hs
Laricifomes officinalis (Vill.: Fr) Kotl. & Pouzar, Ceská Mykol. 3: 158. 1957. G
Boletus purgans Pers., Syn. Meth. Fung. 2: 531. 1801. Hs
Boletus laricis Jacq., Misc. Austriac. 1: 172, t. 20-21. 1778. Hn R

→ **Fomitopsis pinicola** (Sw.: Fr.) P. Karst., Meddeland. Soc. Fauna Fl. Fenn. 6:

9. 1881.
Coriolaceae **POLYP-P**.
Boletus pinicola Sw.: Fr., Kongl. Vetensk. Acad. Nya Handl. 31: 88. 1810.
Polyporus pinicola Sw.: Fr., Syst. Mycol. 1: 372. 1821. Hn R
Polyporus "pinicolus" (Amer Pharm.) is an orthographic variant, Boletus pinus (Amer. Pharm.) cannot be traced. Common homeopathic name: Pine agaric.

Fragaria vesca L., Sp. Pl. 1: 494. 1753.
Rosaceae **FRAG**. Hn R

Franciscaea uniflora see *Brunfelsia uniflora*

Franciscea uniflora see *Brunfelsia uniflora*

Frangula alnus Mill., Gard. Dict. ed. 8. "Frangula" 1. 1768.
Rhamnaceae **RHAM-F**. F
Rhamnus frangula L., Sp. Pl. 1: 193. 1753. Hn R G A F
Frangula vulgaris Hill, Brit. Herb. fasc. 51, 519. 1757. A
Frangula vulgaris Rchb., Fl. Germ. Excurs. 488. 1832. A

Frangula caroliniana see *Rhamnus cathartica*

Frangula vulgaris see *Frangula alnus*

Fraxinus acuminata see *Fraxinus americana*

Fraxinus alba see *Fraxinus americana*

Fraxinus americana L., Sp. Pl. 2: 1057. 1753.
Oleaceae **FRAX**. Hn R A F
Fraxinus alba Marshall, Arbust. Amer. 51. 1785. A F
Fraxinus acuminata Lam., Encycl. 2: 547. 1786. A

Fraxinus excelsior L., Sp. Pl. 2: 1057. 1753.
Oleaceae **FRAX-E**. Hn R F

Fucus helminthochorton see *Alsidium helminthochorton*

Fucus vesiculosus L., Sp. Pl. 2: 1158. 1753.
Fucophyceae **FUC**. Hn R A F

Fumaria fungosa see *Adlumia fungosa*

Fumaria officinalis L., Sp. Pl. 2: 700. 1753.
Fumariaceae **FUM**. Hn R G F

Galanthus nivalis L., Sp. Pl. 1: 288. 1753.
Amaryllidaceae **GALA**. Hn R

Galega officinalis L., Sp. Pl. 2: 714. 1753.
Fabaceae **GALEG**. Hn R G

Galinsoga parviflora Cav., Icon. 3(2): 41, pl. 281. 1795.
Asteraceae **GALIN**. Hn R

Galipea cusparia see *Angostura trifoliata*

Galipea officinalis see *Angostura trifoliata*

Galium aparine L., Sp. Pl. 1: 108. 1753.
Rubiaceae GALI. Hn R G

Galium odoratum (L.) Scop., Fl. Carniol. ed. 1, 105. 1760.
Rubiaceae ASPER. R G
Asperula odorata L., Sp. Pl. 1: 103. 1753. Hn

Galphimia glauca see *Thryallis glauca*

Galphimia gracilis see *Thryallis glauca*

Gambogia see *Garcinia morella*

Garcinia morella Desr., Encycl. 3: 701. 1792.
Clusiaceae GAMB. R A
Common homeopathic name: Gambogia. Several species of *Garcinia*, yeild the resin gamboge.

Gaultheria procumbens L., Sp. Pl. 1: 395. 1753.
Ericaceae GAUL. Hn R G A

Gelsemium nitidum see *Gelsemium sempervirens*

Gelsemium nitidus see *Gelsemium sempervirens*

Gelsemium sempervirens (L.) J. St.-Hil., Expos. Fam. Nat. 1: 338. Feb-Apr 1805.
Loganiaceae GELS. Hn R G A
Bignonia sempervirens L., Sp. Pl. 2: 623. 1753. F
Gelsemium sempervirens (L.) W. T. Aiton, Hortus Kew. 2(2): 64. 1811. nom. illeg., not Pers. 1805 nor J. St.-Hil. 1805. F
Gelsemium sempervirens (L.) Pers., Syn. Pl. 1: 267. Apr-Jun 1805. nom. illeg., not (L.) J. St.-Hil., Feb-Apr 1805.
Gelsemium nitidum Michx., Fl. Bor.-Amer. ed. 1, 1: 120. 1803. A
Gelsemium "nitidus" (Fren. Pharm.) is an orthographic variant.

Genista tinctoria L., Sp. Pl. 2: 710. 1753.
Fabaceae GENIST. Hn R G A

Gentiana cruciata L., Sp. Pl. 1: 231. 1753.
Gentianaceae GENT-C. Hn R A

Gentiana lutea L., Sp. Pl. 1: 227. 1753.
Gentianaceae GENT-L. Hn R G F

Gentiana quinquefolia see *Gentianella quinquefolia*

Gentianella quinquefolia (L.) Small, Fl. S.E. U.S. 929. 1903.
Gentianaceae GENT-Q. Hn R
Gentiana quinquefolia L., Sp. Pl. 1: 230. 1753.

Geranium cicutarium see *Erodium cicutarium*

Geranium emarginatum see *Monsonia emarginata*

Geranium maculatum L., Sp. Pl. 2: 681. 1753.
  Geraniaceae GER. Hn R A
  Incorrect usage: *Geranium pusillum* sensu Germ. and Amer. Pharm., not Burm. f.

Geranium pusillum see *Geranium maculatum*

Geum rivale L., Sp. Pl. 1: 501. 1753.
  Rosaceae GEUM Hn R
  Incorrect usage: *Geum urbanum* sensu Germ. and Amer. Pharm., not L.

Geum urbanum see *Geum rivale*

Ginkgo biloba L., Mant. Pl. 2: 313. 1771.
  Ginkgoaceae GINK. Hn R G F

Ginseng see *Aralia quinquefolia*

Glechoma hederacea L., Sp. Pl. 2: 578. 1753.
  Lamiaceae GLECH. Hn R
  Nepeta hederacea (L.) Trevis., Prosp. Fl. Eugan. 26. 1842. Hs
  Nepeta glechoma Benth., Labiat. Gen. Spec. 485. 1834.

Glycosmis pentaphylla (Retz.) Corrêa, Ann. Mus. Natl. Hist. Nat. 6: 386. 1805.
  Rutaceae ATISTA R
  Limonia pentaphylla Retz., Observ. Bot. 5:. 24. 1789.
  Ghose (1980 p. 176) cites Atista indica (Hom. name) as an alternative name for *Glycosmis pentaphylla*.

Gnaphalium polycephalum Michx., Fl. Bor.-Amer. ed. 1, 2: 127. 1803.
  Asteraceae GNAPH. Hn R A

Gonolobus cundurango see *Marsdenia cundurango*

Gossypium herbaceum L., Sp. Pl. 2: 693. 1753.
  Malvaceae GOSS. Hn R A

Granatum see *Punica granatum*

Gratiola officinalis L., Sp. Pl. 1: 17. 1753.
  Scrophulariaceae GRAT. Hn R G A

Grindelia camporum see *Grindelia rubricaulis* var. *robusta*

Grindelia humilis see *Grindelia rubricaulis* var. *robusta*

Grindelia latifolia see *Grindelia rubricaulis* var. *robusta*

Grindelia robusta see *Grindelia rubricaulis* var. *robusta*

Grindelia rubricaulis DC. var. **robusta** (Nutt.) Steyerm., Ann. Missouri Bot. Gard. 21(1): 227. 1934.
  Asteraceae GRIN.
  Grindelia robusta Nutt., Trans. Amer. Philos. Soc. n.s., 7: 314. 1840. Hn R G A F

A mixture of the different species of *Grindelia* are used by the major pharmacopoeias. These are mainly *Grindelia camporum* Greene, *Grindelia humilis* Hook. & Arn., *Grindelia latifolia* Kellogg, and *Grindelia squarrosa* (Pursh) Dunal.

Grindelia squarrosa see *Grindelia rubricaulis* var. *robusta*

Guaco see *Mikania amara* var. *guaco*

Guaiacum officinale L., Sp. Pl. 1: 381. 1753.
Zygophyllaceae GUAI. Hn R G A F
The dried resin from either *Guaiacum sanctum* L. or *Guaiacum officinale* L. is used for the preparation of the remedy.

Guaiacum sanctum see *Guaiacum officinale*

Guarana see *Paullinia cupana*

Guarea guidonia (L.) Sleumer, Taxon 5: 194. 1956.
Meliaceae GUARE.
Samyda guidonia L., Sp. Pl. 1: 443. 1753.
Guarea trichilioides L., Mant. Pl. 2: 228. 1771, nom. illeg. superfl. Hn R A

Guarea trichilioides see *Guarea guidonia*

Guatteria gaumeri Greenm., Publ. Field Columbian Mus., Bot. ser. 2: 251. 1907.
Annonaceae GUAT.
Guatteria "guameri" (Comp. Rep.) is a typographic error. Dr Gaumer in whose honor the species is named, states that the plant commonly known as "Elemuy" yeilds one of the most valuable medicines used in Yucatan.

Guatteria guameri see *Guatteria gaumeri*

Guilandina bonduc see *Caesalpinia bonduc*

Guilandina dioica see *Gymnocladus dioica*

Gymnema sylvestre (Retz.) R. Br. ex Schult., Syst. Veg. 6: 57. 1820.
Asclepiadaceae GYMNE. Hn R
Periploca sylvestris Retz., Observ. Bot. 2: 15. 1781.

Gymnocladus canadensis see *Gymnocladus dioica*

Gymnocladus dioica (L.) K. Koch, Dendrologic 1: 5. 1869.
Fabaceae GYMN.
Guilandina dioica L., Sp. Pl. 1: 381. 1753. A
Gymnocladus canadensis Lam., Encycl. 1(2): 733. 1785. Hn R A

Haematoxylum campechianum L., Sp. Pl. 1: 384. 1753.
Fabaceae HAEM. Hn R A

Hagenia abyssinica (Bruce) J. F. Gmel., Syst. Nat. ed. 13[bis], 613. 1791.
Rosaceae KOU.
Bankesia abbyssinica Bruce, Select Spec. Nat. Hist. 73. 1790.
Brayera anthelmintica Kunth, Bull. Sci. Soc. Philom. Paris 154. 1822. R

Common homeopathic name: Kousso.

Hamamelis dioica see *Hamamelis virginiana*

Hamamelis macrophylla see *Hamamelis virginiana*

Hamamelis virginiana L., Sp. Pl. 1: 124. 1753.
Hamamelidaceae HAM. R G A F
Hamamelis macrophylla Pursh, Fl. Amer. Sept. 1: 116. 1814. Hn A
Hamamelis dioica Walter, Fl. Carol. 255. 1788. A

Haplopappus baylahuen Remy, Fl. Chil. 4(1): 42. 1849.
Asteraceae HAPL-B. Hn R G

Harpagophytum procumbens DC. ex Meisn., Pl. Vasc. Gen. 1: 298, 2: 206. 1840.
Pedaliceae HARP. Hn R G F

Harrisia bonplandii (Parm. ex Pfeiff.) Britton & Rose, Cact. 2: 157. 1920.
Cactaceae CERE-B. R
Cereus bonplandii Parm. ex Pfeiff., Enum. Diagn. Cact. 108. 1837. Hn A
Incorrect usage: *Cactus bonplandii* sensu Amer. Pharm., not Kunth.

Hedeoma pulegioides (L.) Pers., Syn. Pl. 2: 131. 1806.
Lamiaceae HEDEO. Hn R A
Cunila pulegioides L., Sp. Pl. ed. 2. 30. 1762. A

Hedera helix L., Sp. Pl. 1: 202. 1753.
Araliaceae HED. Hn R G A F

Hedera quinquefolia see *Parthenocissus quinquefolia*

Hedysarum barbatum see *Desmodium barbatum*

Hedysarum desmodium see *Desmodium barbatum*

Hedysarum gangeticum see *Desmodium gangeticum*

Hedysarum Ildefonsianum see *Desmodium barbatum*

Hedysarum lagocephalum see *Desmodium barbatum*

Helianthemum canadense (L.) Michx., Fl. Bor.-Amer. ed. 1, 1: 308. 1803.
Cistaceae CIST. Hs
Cistus canadensis L., Sp. Pl. 1: 526. 1753. Hn R A
Incorrect usage: *Cistus helianthemum* sensu Amer. Pharm., not L.

Helianthus annuus L., Sp. Pl. 2: 904. 1753.
Asteraceae HELIA. Hn R G A F

Heliotropium arborescens L., Sp. Pl. ed. 2, 1: 187. 1762.
Boraginaceae HELIO.
Heliotropium peruvianum L., Sp. Pl. ed. 2, 1: 187. 1762. Hn R A

Heliotropium peruvianum see *Heliotropium arborescens*

Helleborus foetidus L., Sp. Pl. 1: 558. 1753.

Ranunculaceae HELL-F. Hn R A

Helleborus grandiflorus see *Helleborus niger*

Helleborus hyemalis see *Eranthis hyemalis*

Helleborus niger L., Sp. Pl. 1: 558. 1753.
Ranunculaceae HELL. Hn R A F
Helleborus grandiflorus Salisb., Prodr. Stirp. Chap. Allerton 374. 1796. A
Incorrect usage: *Veratrum nigrum* sensu Amer. Pharm., not L.

Helleborus orientalis Lam., Encycl. 3: 96. 1789.
Ranunculaceae HELL-O. R

Helleborus viridis L., Sp. Pl. 1: 558. 1753.
Ranunculaceae HELL-V. Hn R

Helmintochortos see *Alsidium helminthochorton*

Helonias dioica (Walter) Pursh, Fl. Amer. Sept. 1: 243. 1814.
Melanthiaceae HELON. Hn R A
Melanthium dioicum Walter, Fl. Carol. 126. 1788. A
Incorrect usage: *Chamaelirium luteum* sensu Germ. and Amer. Pharm., not (L.) A. Gray; *Veratrum luteum* (Hom. syn.) not L. and *Helonias lutea* (Amer. Pharm., and Hom. syn.) not Ker-Gawl.

Helonias lutea see *Helonias dioica*

Helonias viridis (Aiton) Ker Gawl., Bot. Mag. 27: t. 1096. 1808.
Melanthiaceae VERAT-V. A
Veratrum viride Aiton, Hort. Kew. 3: 422. 1789. Hn R A
The only evidence that Ker-Gawl is the authority for *Helonias viridis*, is through the cross reference to *Helonias virginica* (Bot. Mag. t. 985. 1808), which is clearly written by "G".

Hepatica nobilis Mill., Gard. Dict. ed. 8. "Hepatica" 1. 1768.
Ranunculaceae HEPAT.
Hepatica triloba Chaix, Hist. Pl. Dauphiné 1: 336. 1786. Hn R A
Anemone hepatica L., Sp. Pl. 1: 538. 1753. A

Hepatica triloba see *Hepatica nobilis*

Heracleum sphondylium L., Sp. Pl. 1: 249. 1753.
Apiaceae BRAN. R A F
Branca ursina (Amer. Pharm., and Hom. name) is a pre-Linnaean name.

Hibiscus abelmoschus see *Abelmoschus moschatus*

Hieracium pilosella L. Sp. Pl. 2: 800. 1753.
Asteraceae HIER-P. Hn R F

Hippomane mancinella L., Sp. Pl. 2: 1191. 1753.
Euphorbiaceae MANC. R A
Common homeopathic name: Mancinella.

Hoang-nan see *Strychnos axillaris*

Hoitzia coccina see *Loeselia coccinea*

Hoitzia coccinea see *Loeselia coccinea*

Holarrhena antidysenterica see *Holarrhena pubescens*

Holarrhena pubescens (Buch.-Ham.) Wall. ex G. Don., Gen. Hist. 4(1): 78. 1837.
Apocynaceae KURCH.
Echites pubescens Buch.-Ham., Trans. Linn. Soc. London 13(2): 524. 1822.
Holarrhena antidysenterica (L.) Wall. ex A. DC., Prodr. 8: 413. Mar 1844. R
Echites antidysenterica Roth, Syst. Veg. 4: 394. 1819.
Echites antidysenterica (L.) Roxb. ex Fleming, Asiat. Res. 11: 166. 1810.
Common homeopathic name: Kurchi bark.

Homeria breyniana (L.) G. J. Lewis, J. S. African Bot. 7: 59. 1941.
Iridaceae HOME.
Tulipa breyniana L., Sp. Pl. 1: 306. 1753.
Homeria collina (Thunb.) Vent., Dec. Gen. Nov. 5. 1808. Hn R

Homeria collina see *Homeria breyniana*

Humulus lupulus L., Sp. Pl. 2: 1028. 1753.
Cannabaceae LUP. R G A F
Lupulus humulus (Hom. name) is a nom. nud.

Hura brasiliensis see *Hura crepitans*

Hura crepitans L., Sp. Pl. 2: 1008. 1753.
Euphorbiaceae HURA-C. Hn R
Hura brasiliensis Willd., Enum. Pl. 997. 1809. Hn R
Hura brasiliensis (Comp. Rep.) is cited as a separate remedy, with the abbreviation HURA.

Hyacinthoides non-scripta (L.) Chouard ex Rothm., Feddes Repert. 53: 14. 1944.
Hyacinthaceae AGRA. F
Hyacinthus non-scriptus L., Sp. Pl. 1: 316. 1753.
Scilla nutans Sm., Engl. Bot. 6: pl. 377. 1797. R
Agraphis nutans Link, Handbuch. 1: 166. 1829. Hn F

Hyacinthus non-scriptus see *Hyacinthoides non-scripta*

Hydnocarpus kurzii (King) Warb., Nat. Pflanzenfam. 3(6a): 21. 1893.
Flacourtiaceae CHAUL. R
Taraktogenos kurzii King, J. Asiat. Soc. Bengal, Pt. 2, Nat. Hist. 59: 123. 1890.
Common homeopathic name: Chaulmoogra.

Hydrangea arborescens L., Sp. Pl. 1: 397. 1753.
Hydrangeaceae HYDRANG. Hn R A

Hydrastis canadensis L., Syst. Nat. ed. 10, 2: 1088. 1759.
Ranunculaceae HYDR. Hn R G A F

Warneria canadensis Mill., Fig. Pl. Gard. Dict. t. 285. 1755. A

Hydrocotyl nummariodes see *Centella asiatica*

Hydrocotyle asiatica see *Centella asiatica*

Hydrocotyle nummularioides see *Centella asiatica*

Hydrophyllum virginianum L., Sp. Pl. 1: 146. 1753.
Hydrophyllaceae HYDRO-V. Hn R A

Hylotelephium telephium (L.) Ohba, Bot. Mag. (Tokyo) 90(1017): 53. 1977.
Crassulaceae SED-T.
Sedum telephium L., Sp. Pl. 1: 430. 1753. Hn R

Hyoscyamus lethalis see *Hyoscyamus niger*

Hyoscyamus niger L., Sp. Pl. 1: 179. 1753.
Solanaceae HYOS. Hn R G A F
Hyoscyamus vulgaris Bubani, Fl. Pyren. 1: 351. 1897.
Hyoscyamus vulgaris Neck., Delic. Gallo-Belg. 1: 122. 1768. A
Hyoscyamus lethalis Salisb., Prodr. Stirp. Chap. Allerton 131. 1796. A

Hyoscyamus vulgaris see *Hyoscyamus niger*

Hypericum perforatum L., Sp. Pl. 2: 785. 1753.
Clusiaceae HYPER. Hn R G A F

Hypopterygium adstringens see *Amphipterygium adstringens*

Iberis amara L., Sp. Pl. 2: 649. 1753.
Brassicaceae IBER. Hn R G A F
Incorrect usage: *Lepidium iberis* sensu Amer. Pharm., not L.

Ictodes foetida see *Symplocarpus foetidus*

Ictodes foetidus see *Symplocarpus foetidus*

Ignatia amara see *Strychnos ignatii*

Ilex aquifolium L., Sp. Pl. 1: 125. 1753.
Aquifoliaceae ILX-A. Hn R G A
Incorrect usage: *Ilex opaca* sensu Amer. Pharm., not Sol., and *Ilex canadensis* sensu Amer. Pharm., not Marsh.

Ilex canadensis see *Ilex aquifolium*

Ilex cassine L., Sp. Pl. 1: 125. 1753.
Aquifoliaceae ILX-C. Hn R

Ilex mate see *Ilex paraguariensis*

Ilex opaca see *Ilex aquifolium*

Ilex paraguariensis A. St.-Hil., Mem. Mus. Paraná 9: 351. 1822.
Aquifoliaceae MATE R
Ilex paraguensis D. Don, Descr. Pinus ed. 2, 2: 49. t. 11. 1828. A
Ilex paraguayensis Hook., Bot. Mag. 69. t. 3992. 1843. A

Annotated Checklist

Ilex mate A. St.-Hil., Pl. Rem. 1: 41. 1824. {Publication not seen} A
Common homeopathic name: Maté.

Ilex paraguayensis see *Ilex paraguariensis*

Ilex paraguensis see *Ilex paraguariensis*

Illecebrum achyrantha see *Alternanthera repens*

Illicium anisatum L., Syst. Nat. ed. 10, 2: 1050. 1759.
Illiciaceae ANIS. Hs
Incorrect usage: *Illicium verum* sensu Comp. Rep., and Amer. Pharm., not Hook. f. Linnaeus (1749 p. 180) uses Anisum stellatum (Hom. name) as the medicinal name.

Illicium verum see *Illicium anisatum*

Imperatoria ostruthium see *Peucedanum ostruthium*

Indigofera indica see *Indigofera tinctoria*

Indigofera tinctoria L., Sp. Pl. 2: 751. 1753.
Fabaceae INDG. Hn R A
Indigofera indica Lam. Encycl. 3(1): 245. 1789, nom. illeg., not Mill. 1768. A

Inula helenium L., Sp. Pl. 2: 881. 1753.
Asteraceae INUL. Hn R A

Ipecacuanha see *Psychotria ipecacuanha*

Ipomoea alba L., Sp. Pl. 1: 161. 1753.
Convolvulaceae CONVO-D.
Ipomoea bona-nox L., Sp. Pl. ed. 2, 1: 228. 1762. R A
Convolvulus pulcherrimus Vell., Fl. Flumin. 1: 72. t. 54. 1825. A
Calonyction speciosum Choisy, Convolv. Orient. 59. 1834. A
Convolvulus duartinus (Hom. name) is cited by Grieve (1931 p. 103) as an alternative name for *Ipomoea bona-nox*.

Ipomoea bona-nox see *Ipomoea alba*

Ipomoea jalapa see *Ipomoea purga*

Ipomoea purga (Wender.) Hayne, Getreue Darstell. Gew. Bd. 12: 5, t. 33 & 34. 1833.
Convolvulaceae JAL. R A
Convolvulus purga Wender., Pharm. Central-Blatt 1: 457. 1830. Hs
Ipomoea jalapa Schiede & Deppe ex G. Don Gen. Hist. 4(1): 271. 1837, not (L.) Pursh 1813. A
Exogonium purga (Wender.) Benth., Pl. Hartw. 46. 1840.
Incorrect usage: *Convolvulus jalapa* sensu Amer. Pharm., not L. Common homeopathic name: Jalapa.

Ipomoea purpurea (L.) Roth, Bot. Abh. Beobacht. 27. 1787.
Convolvulaceae IPOM. Hn R
Convolvulus purpureus L., Sp. Pl. ed. 2. 1: 219. 1762.

Ipomoea turpethum see *Operculina turpethum*

Iresine calea (Ibáñez) Standl., Contr. U. S. Natl. Herb. 18(3): 94. 1916.
Amaranthaceae ACHY.
Achyranthes calea Ibáñez, Naturaleza (Mexico City) 4: 79. 1877. Hn R A

Iris florentina L., Syst. Nat. ed. 10, 2: 863. 1759.
Iridaceae IRIS-FL. Hn R

Iris foetidissima L., Sp. Pl. 1: 39. 1753.
Iridaceae IRIS-FOE. Hn R

Iris germanica L., Sp. Pl. 1: 38. 1753.
Iridaceae IRIS-G. Hn R

Iris minor see *Iris tenax*

Iris tenax Douglas ex Lindl., Bot. Reg. 15: t. 1218. 1829.
Iridaceae IRIS-T. Hn R
Iris minor (Hom. syn.) is cited by Grieve (1931 p. 439) as an alternative name for *Iris tenax*.

Iris versicolor L., Sp. Pl. 1: 39. 1753.
Iridaceae IRIS Hn R G A F

Jaborandi see *Pilocarpus microphyllus*

Jacaranda caroba (Vell.) DC., Prodr. 9: 232. Jan 1845.
Bignoniaceae JAC-C. Hn R A
Bignonia caroba Vell., Fl. Flumin. 250. 1829. Hs A

Jacaranda gualandai see *Jacaranda mimosifolia*

Jacaranda gualanday see *Jacaranda mimosifolia*

Jacaranda mimosifolia D. Don, Bot. Reg. 8: pl. 631. 1822.
Bignoniaceae JAC.
Jacaranda gualanday Cortés, Fl. Colombia. 99. 1897, nom. nud.
Jacaranda "gualandai" (Comp. Rep.) is a typographic error.

Jalapa see *Ipomoea purga*

Jambos vulgaris see *Syzygium jambos*

Jasminum officinale L., Sp. Pl. 1: 7. 1753.
Oleaceae JASM. Hn R

Jatropha curcas L., Sp. Pl. 2: 1006. 1753.
Euphorbiaceae JATR. Hn R A
Curcas purgans Medik., Malvenfam. 119. 1787. A
Castiglionia lobata Ruiz & Pav., Fl. Peruv. 1: 277. 1798. A

Jatropha urens see *Cnidoscolus urens*

Joanesia asoca see *Saraca asoca*

Juglans cathartica see *Juglans cinerea*

Juglans cinerea L., Syst. Nat. ed. 10, 2: 1272. 1759.
Juglandaceae JUG-C. Hn R A
Juglans cathartica F. Michx., Hist. Arbr. Forest. 1: 165. 1810, incertae sedis. A

Juglans regia L., Sp. Pl. 2: 997. 1753.
Juglandaceae JUG-R. Hn R A

Juglans tomentosa see *Carya tomentosa*

Juliana adstringens see *Amphipterygium adstringens*

Juliania adstringens see *Amphipterygium adstringens*

Juncus communis see *Juncus effusus*

Juncus effusus L., Sp. Pl. 1: 326. 1753.
Juncaceae JUNC. Hn R A
Juncus communis E. Mey., Junc. Monogr. Spec. 12. 1819. A

Juniperus communis L., Sp. Pl. 2: 1040. 1753.
Cupressaceae JUNI-C. Hn R G F

Juniperus foetida see *Juniperus sabina*

Juniperus sabina L., Sp. Pl. 2: 1039. 1753.
Cupressaceae SABIN. R Hs G A
Sabina officinalis Garcke, Fl. N. Mitt.-Deutschland ed. 4, 387. 1858.
Incorrect usage: *Juniperus foetida* sensu Amer. Pharm., not Spach. Linnaeus (1749 p. 165) uses Sabina (Hom. name) as the medicinal name for *Juniperus sabina*.

Juniperus virginiana L., Sp. Pl. 2: 1039. 1753.
Cupressaceae JUNI-V. Hn R A

Justicia adhatoda see *Adhatoda vasica*

Justicia paniculata see *Andrographis paniculata*

Justicia rubra see *Odontonema rubrum*

Justicia rubrum see *Odontonema rubrum*

Kalmia latifolia L., Sp. Pl. 1: 391. 1753.
Ericaceae KALM. Hn R G A F

Kamala see *Mallotus philippensis*

Karaka see *Corynocarpus laevigatus*

Karwinskia humboldtiana (Roem. & Schult.) Zucc., Abh. Math.-Phys. Cl. Königl. Bayer. Akad. Wiss. 1: 353. 1832.
Rhamnaceae KARW-H. Hn R A
Rhamnus humboldtiana Roem. & Schult., Syst. Veg. 5: 295. 1819.

Kola see *Cola acuminata*

Kousso see *Hagenia abyssinica*

Krameria lappacea (Dombey) Burdet & Simpson, Candollea 38: 696. 1983.
Krameriaceae RAT.
Landia lappacea Dombey, J. Sçavans (Paris, 12°) 1: 382. 1784. {Publication not seen}
Krameria triandra Ruiz & Pav., Fl. Peruv. 1: 33. 1798. R G A F
Ratanhia peruviana, (Hom. name, Amer., Fren., and Germ. Pharm.) is a nom. nud. Simpson (Candollea 38: 46.1983) cites *Krameria lappacea* as constituting the true 'rhatany' of commerce.

Krameria triandra see *Krameria lappacea*

Kurchi see *Holarrhena pubescens*

Laburnum anagyroides Medik., Vorles. Churpfälz. Phys.-Öcon. Ges. 2: 363. 1787.
Fabaceae CYT-L. R G A
Cytisus laburnum L., Sp. Pl. 2: 739. 1753. Hn A

Lachnanthes caroliniana (Lam.) Dandy, J. Bot. 70: 329. 1932.
Haemodoraceae LACHN.
Dilatris caroliniana Lam., Tabl. Encycl. 1: 127. 1791. A
Lachnanthes tinctoria (Walter ex J. F. Gmel.) Elliott, Sketch Bot. S. Carolina 1(1): 47. 1816. Hn R A

Lachnanthes tinctoria see *Lachnanthes caroliniana*

Lactuca sinuata see *Lactuca virosa*

Lactuca virosa L., Sp. Pl. 2: 795. 1753.
Asteraceae LACT. Hn R A
Lactuca sinuata Forssk., Fl. Aegypt.-Arab. 215. 1775, incertae sedis. A

Lamium album L., Sp. Pl. 2: 579. 1753.
Lamiaceae LAM. Hn R G A F
Incorrect usage: *Lamium maculatum* (Hom. syn., and Amer. Pharm.) not L.

Lamium laevigatum auct.

Lamium laevigatum see *Lamium album*

Lamium maculatum see *Lamium album*

Landia lappacea see *Krameria lappacea*

Lapathum see *Rumex obtusifolius*

Laportea crenulata see *Dendrocnide sinuata*

Laportea gigas Wedd., Nouv. Arch. Mus. Hist. Nat. 9: 1-400. 1856, 401-591. 1857.
Urticaceae URT-G. R
Urtica gigas A. Cunn. ex Heward, J. Bot. (Hooker) 4. 292. 1841. Hn

Lappa arctium see *Arctium lappa*

Lappa major see *Arctium lappa*

Lapsana communis L., Sp. Pl. 2: 811. 1753.
   Asteraceae LAPS. Hn R

Laricifomes officinalis see *Fomitopsis officinalis*

Larrea mexicana see *Larrea tridentata*

Larrea tridentata (Sessé & Moç. ex DC.) Coville, Contr. U. S. Natl. Herb. 4: 75. 1893.
   Zygophyllaceae PALO.
   Zygophyllum tridentatum Sessé & Moç. ex DC., Prodr. 1: 706. Jan 1824. Hs
   Larrea mexicana Moric., Pl. Nouv. Amér. 71. pl. 48. 1839. R
   Paloondo (Hom. name) is the vernacular name.

Lathyrus sativus L., Sp. Pl. 2: 730. 1753.
   Fabaceae LATH. Hn R A

Laurocerasus officinalis see *Prunus laurocerasus*

Laurus benzoin see *Lindera benzoin*

Laurus camphora see *Cinnamomum camphora*

Laurus cassia see *Cinnamomum zeylanicum*

Laurus cinnamomum see *Cinnamomum zeylanicum*

Ledum palustre L., Sp. Pl. 1: 391. 1753.
   Ericaceae LED. Hn R G A F

Lemna minor L., Sp. Pl. 2: 970. 1753.
   Lemnaceae LEM-M. Hn R G

Leontice thalictroides see *Caulophyllum thalictroides*

Leontodon taraxacum see *Taraxacum officinale*

Leonurus cardiaca L., Sp. Pl. 2: 584. 1753.
   Lamiaceae LEON. Hn R G

Lepidium bonariense L., Sp. Pl. 2: 645. 1753.
   Brassicaceae LEPI. Hn R

Lepidium iberis see *Iberis amara*

Lepiota procera see *Macrolepiota procera*

Leptandra virginica see *Veronicastrum virginicum*

Leucanthemum vulgare Lam., Fl. Franç. 2: 137. 1778.
   Asteraceae CHRYSAN. R
   Chrysanthemum leucanthemum L., Sp. Pl. 2: 888. 1753. Hn

Liatris spicata (L.) Willd., Willd., Sp. Pl. 3(3): 1636. 1803.
   Asteraceae LIATR. Hn R
   Serratula spicata L., Sp. Pl. 2: 819. 1753.

Lichen barbatus see *Usnea barbata*

Lichen islandicus see *Cetraria islandica*

Lichen pulmonarius see *Lobaria pulmonaria*

Lilium lancifolium Thunb., Trans. Linn. Soc. London 2: 333. 1794.
Liliaceae LIL-T. Hs G
Lilium tigrinum Ker Gawl., Bot. Mag. 31: t. 1237. 1809. Hn R A F

Lilium superbum L., Sp. Pl. ed. 2, 1: 434. 1762.
Liliaceae LIL-S. Hn R

Lilium tigrinum see *Lilium lancifolium*

Limonia pentaphylla see *Glycosmis pentaphylla*

Linaria vulgaris Mill., Gard. Dict. ed. 8. "Linaria" 1. 1768.
Scrophulariaceae LINA. Hn R A
Antirrhinum linaria L., Sp. Pl. 2: 616. 1753.
Antirrhinum "linarium" (Amer. Pharm.) is an orthographic variant.

Lindera benzoin (L.) Blume, Mus. Bot. 1: 324. 1851.
Lauraceae BENZO. R
Laurus benzoin L., Sp. Pl. 1: 370. 1753. Hs
Linnaeus (1749 p. 66) uses Benzoin (Hom. name) as the medicinal name for *Laurus benzoin*.

Linum catharticum L., Sp. Pl. 1: 281. 1753.
Linaceae LINU-C. Hn R A

Linum usitatissimum L., Sp. Pl. 1: 277. 1753.
Linaceae LINU-U. Hn R

Lippia dulcis see *Phyla scaberrima*

Lippia mexicana see *Phyla scaberrima*

Lithospermum virginianum see *Onosmodium virginianum*

Lobaria pulmonaria (L.) Hoffm., Deutschl. Fl. 146. 1796.
Lobariaceae STICT. G A F
Lichen pulmonarius L., Sp. Pl. 2: 1145. 1753.
Sticta pulmonaria Hook., Fl. Scot. 58. 1821. Hn R A
Sticta pulmonacea Ach., Lichenogr. universalis 449. 1810.
Parmelia pulmonacea (L.) Biroli, Fl. Acon. 2: 188. 1808.
Sticta "pulmonaceae" (Fren. Pharm.) is a typographic error.

Lobelia cardinalis L., Sp. Pl. 2: 930. 1753.
Campanulaceae LOB-C. Hn R A

Lobelia colorata Wall., Pl. Asiat. Rar. 2: 42. 1831.
Campanulaceae LOB-P. Hs
Lobelia purpurascens Wall., Numer. List n. 1307. 1829, nom. nud. Hn R

Lobelia dortmanna L., Sp. Pl. 2: 929. 1753.
Campanulaceae LOB-D. Hn R

Lobelia erinus L., Sp. Pl. 2: 932. 1753.
Campanulaceae LOB-E. Hn R

Lobelia inflata L., Sp. Pl. 2: 931. 1753.
Campanulaceae LOB. Hn R G A

Lobelia purpurascens see *Lobelia colorata*

Lobelia siphilitica L., Sp. Pl. 2: 931. 1753.
Campanulaceae LOB-S. Hn R A

Lodoicea maldivica (J. F. Gmelin) Pers., Syn. Pl. 2: 630. 1807.
Arecaceae NUX-A.
Cocos maldivica J. F. Gmelin, Syst. Nat. 2(1): 569. 1791, ("maldioica" - corrected 1796).
Also see Sonnerat for informal description. The homeopathic name Nux absurda cannot be traced and is probably trivial.

Loeselia coccina see *Loeselia coccinea*

Loeselia coccinea (Cav.) G. Don, Gen. Hist. 4(2): 247. 1838.
Polemoniaceae HOIT.
Hoitzia coccinea Cav., Icon. 4: 44, t. 365. 1798. A
Loeselia "coccina" (Comp. Rep., and Hom. name) is a typographic error.

Lolium robustum see *Lolium temulentum*

Lolium temulentum L., Sp. Pl. 1: 83. 1753.
Poaceae LOL. Hn R A
Lolium robustum Rchb., Icon. Pl. Germ. Helv. 1: t. 4. f. 1340. 1834-1836. A

Lonicera alba see *Chiococca alba*

Lonicera caprifolium L., Sp. Pl. 1: 173. 1753.
Caprifoliaceae LON-C. Hn R F

Lonicera marilandica see *Spigelia marilandica*

Lonicera periclymenum L., Sp. Pl. 1: 173. 1753.
Caprifoliaceae LON-P. Hn R

Lonicera xylosteum L., Sp. Pl. 1: 174. 1753.
Caprifoliaceae LON-X. Hn R

Lophophora williamsii (Lem.) J.M. Coult. var. **lewinii** J. M. Coult., Contr. U.S. Natl. Herb. 3: 131. 1894.
Cactaceae ANH. R A
Anhalonium lewinii Hennings ex Lewin, Gartenflora 37: 410. 1888. Hn A

Lophophytum leandri see *Lophophytum leandrii*

Lophophytum leandrii Eichler, Fl. Bras. 4(2): 59, t. 15. 1869.
Balanophoraceae FLOR-P.
Flor de piedra (Hom. name) appears to be the vernacular name. *Lophophytum "leandri"* (Comp. Rep.) is a typographic error.

Luffa amara Roxb., Hort. Bengal. 70. 1814; Fl. Ind. ed. 1832. 3: 715.1832.
Cucurbitaceae LUF-A. Hn R

Luffa bendaul see *Luffa bondel*

Luffa bindaal see *Luffa bondel*

Luffa bondel Buch.-Ham. ex Steud., Nomencl. Bot. ed. 2, 2: 77. 1840.
Cucurbitaceae LUF-B.
Luffa bindal (Comp. Rep.) appears to be a typographic error, the nearest combination is *Luffa bondel*. *Luffa bindaal* is a nom. nud., and is cited as an orthographic variant of *Luffa bendaul* Roxb.

Luffa operculata (L.) Cogn., Fl. Bras. 6(4): 12, pl. 1. 1878.
Cucurbitaceae LUF-OP. Hn R G
Momordica operculata L., Syst. Nat. ed. 10, 1278. 1759.

Luma chequen (Molina) A. Gray, U. S. Expl. Exped., Phan. 536. 1854, "cheken".
Myrtaceae MYRT-CH.
Eugenia chequen Molina, Sag. Stor. Nat. Chili. ed. 2, 148, 289. 1810, "cheken". R
Myrtus chequen (Molina) Spreng., Syst. Veg. 2: 485. 1825.
Myrtus cheken (Hom. name) is an orthographic variant.

Lupulus humulus see *Humulus lupulus*

Lycoperdon bovista see *Calvatia gigantea*

Lycoperdon gigantea see *Calvatia gigantea*

Lycopersicon esculentum see *Solanum lycopersicum*

Lycopersicon lycopersicum see *Solanum lycopersicum*

Lycopodium clavatum L., Sp. Pl. 2: 1101. 1753.
Lycopodiaceae LYC. Hn R G A F

Lycopus europaeus see *Lycopus virginicus*

Lycopus virginicus L., Sp. Pl. 1: 21. 1753.
Lamiaceae LYCPS. Hn R G A F
The French pharmacopoeia uses either *Lycopus europaeus* L. or *Lycopus virginicus* L.

Lysimachia nummularia L., Sp. Pl. 1: 148. 1753.
Primulaceae LYSIM. Hn R

Macaglia quebracho-blanco (Schltdl.) A. Lyons, Pl. Nam. ed 2, 286. 1907.
Apocynaceae QUEB.
Aspidosperma quebracho-blanco Schltdl., Bot. Zeitung (Berlin) 19: 137. 1861.
Aspidosperma quebracho (Comp. Rep.) is not a valid combination. Common homeopathic name: Quebracho.

Macrolepiota procera (Scop.: Fr.) Singer, Pap. Michigan Acad. Sci. 32: 141.

1946 (Publ. 1948).
Agaricaceae AGAR-PR.
Agaricus procerus Scop.: Fr., Fl. Carniol. ed. 2, 2: 418. 1772; Syst. Mycol. 1: 20. 1821. Hn R
Lepiota procera (Scop.: Fr.) Gray, Nat. Arr. Brit. Pl. 1: 601. 1821.
Agaricus procerus Schaeff., Fung. Bavar. Palat. Nasc. 1: 12, t. 23. 1762. Hn R

Macropiper methysticum see *Piper methysticum*

Macrozamia spiralis (Salisb. ex C. W. Konig & Sims) Miq. Monogr. Cycad. 36, t. 4, 5. 1842.
Zamiaceae MACROZ. Hn R
Zamia spiralis Salisb. ex C. W. Konig & Sims, Prodr. Stirp. Chap. Allerton 401. 1796.

Magnolia glauca see *Magnolia virginiana*

Magnolia grandiflora L., Syst. Nat. ed. 10, 2: 1082. 1759.
Magnoliaceae MAGN-GR. Hn R

Magnolia virginiana L., Sp. Pl. 1: 535. 1753.
Magnoliaceae MAGN-GL. R
Magnolia glauca (L.) L., Syst. Nat. ed. 10, 2: 1082. 1759. Hn

Mahonia aquifolium (Pursh) Nutt., Gen. N. Amer. Pl. 1: 212. 1818.
Berberidaceae BERB-A. G F
Berberis aquifolium Pursh, Fl. Amer. Sept. 1: 219, t. 4. 1814. Hn R A

Mallotus philippensis (Lam.) Müll. Arg., Linnaea 34: 196. 1865.
Euphorbiaceae KAM. R
Croton philippensis Lam., Encycl. 2: 206. 1786.
Rottlera tinctoria Roxb., Pl. Coromandel 2: 36, t. 168. 1798. Hs
Croton coccineus Vahl, Symb. Bot. 2: 97. 1791, nom. illeg. Hs
Common homeopathic name: Kamala.

Malosma laurina (Nutt.) Nutt. ex Engl., Monogr. Phan. 4: 393. 1883.
Anacardiaceae RHUS-L.
Rhus laurina Nutt., Fl. N. Amer. 1(2): 219. 1838. Hn R

Malus pumila Mill., Gard. Dict. ed. 8. "Malus" 3. 1768.
Rosaceae PYRUS-M.
Pyrus malus L., Sp. Pl. 1: 479. 1753. Hn
Malus sylvestris Mill., Gard. Dict. ed. 8. "Malus" 1. 1768. R

Malus sylvestris see *Malus pumila*

Manchineel see *Hippomane mancinella*

Mancinella see *Hippomane mancinella*

Mandragora officinarum L., Sp. Pl. 1: 181. 1753.
Solanaceae MAND. Hn R G A

Mangifera indica L., Sp. Pl. 1: 200. 1753.

Anacardiaceae MANGI. Hn R

Manihot esculenta Crantz, Inst. Rei Herb. 1: 167. 1766.
Euphorbiaceae CASS.
Manihot utilissima Pohl, Pl. Bras. Icon. Descr. 1: 32, t. 24. 1827. R
Common homeopathic name: Cassava.

Manihot utilissima see *Manihot esculenta*

Manzanita see *Arctostaphylos pungens*

Marrubium vulgare L., Sp. Pl. 2: 583. 1753.
Lamiaceae MARR. Hn R G

Marsdenia condurango see *Marsdenia cundurango*

Marsdenia cundurango Rchb. f., Bot. Zeitung (Berlin) 30: 552. 1872.
Asclepiadaceae CUND. G
Gonolobus cundurango Triana, Compt. Rend. Hebd. Séances Acad. Sci. 74: 883. 1872. R A
Incorrect author citation: Marsdenia condurango Nichols., (Fren. Pharm.).
Common homeopathic name: Cundurango.

Marum verum see *Teucrium marum*

Mate see *Ilex paraguariensis*

Matico see *Piper aduncum*

Matricaria chamomilla see *Matricaria recutita*

Matricaria parthenium see *Tanacetum parthenium*

Matricaria recutita (L.) Rauschert, Folia Geobot. Phytotax. 9: 254. 1974.
Asteraceae CHAM. F
Matricaria recutita L., Sp. Pl. 2: 891. 1753.
Matricaria chamomilla L., Sp. Pl. ed. 2, 2: 1256. 1763.
Matricaria chamomilla L., Fl. Suec. ed. 2, 296. 1755, not L. 1753. R A F
Chamomilla recutita (L.) Rauschert, Folia Geobot. Phytotax. 9: 254. 1974. G F
Anthemis vulgaris L. ex Steud., Nomencl. Bot. ed. 1(1): 53. 1821. A
Common homeopathic name: Chamomilla.

Matthiola incana (L.) R. Br., Hortus Kew. 4: 119. 1812.
Brassicaceae MATTH. Hn R
Cheiranthus incanus L., Sp. Pl. 2: 662. 1753.

Medicago sativa L., Sp. Pl. 2: 778. 1753.
Fabaceae ALF. R A F
Common homeopathic name: Alfalfa.

Melaleuca cajuputi Powell, Pharm. Roy. Coll. Physic. London (Transl.) 22. 1809, not Roxb. 1814.
Myrtaceae CAJ. R
Incorrect usage: *Melaleuca leucadendron* sensu Amer. Pharm., and Hom.

syn., not *Melaleuca leucadendra* (L.) L. Common homeopathic name: Cajuputum.

Melaleuca leucadendra see *Melaleuca cajuputi*

Melaleuca leucadendron see *Melaleuca cajuputi*

Melanthium dioicum see *Helonias dioica*

Melia azadirachta see *Azadirachta indica*

Melilotus alba see *Melilotus albus*

Melilotus albus Medik., Vorles. Churpfälz. Phys.-Öcon. Ges. 2: 382. 1787.
Fabaceae MELI-A.
Melilotus vulgaris Willd., Enum. Pl. 790. 1809. A
Melilotus leucanthus W. D. J. Koch ex DC., Fl. Franç. Reissue 564. 1815. {Publication not seen}
Melilotus alba Medik., Encycl. 4(1): 63-64. 1797. Desr. is not the correct author see Terrell *et al.* 1989. R
Melilotus "leucantha" (Amer. Pharm.) is an orthographic variant.

Melilotus leucantha see *Melilotus albus*

Melilotus leucanthus see *Melilotus albus*

Melilotus officinalis (L.) Pall., Reise Russ. Reich. 3: 537. 1776.
Fabaceae MELI. Hn R G A F
Trifolium melilotus L. var. *officinalis* L., Sp. Pl. 2: 765. 1753.
Trifolium officinale L., Sp. Pl. 2: 765. 1753. A

Melilotus vulgaris see *Melilotus albus*

Menispermum angulatum see *Menispermum canadense*

Menispermum canadense L., Sp. Pl. 1: 340. 1753.
Menispermaceae MENIS. Hn R A
Menispermum angulatum Moench, Methodus 277. 1794. A

Menispermum cocculus see *Anamirta cocculus*

Menispermum cordifolium see *Tinospora cordifolia*

Mentha officinalis see *Mentha x piperita*

Mentha pulegium L., Sp. Pl. 2: 577. 1753.
Lamiaceae MENTH-PU. Hn R

Mentha spicata L., Sp. Pl. 2: 576. 1753.
Lamiaceae MENTH-V. Hn R
Mentha viridis (L.) L., Sp. Pl. ed. 2, 804. 1763. Hs

Mentha viridis see *Mentha spicata*

Mentha x piperita L., Sp. Pl. 2: 576. 1753.
Lamiaceae MENTH. Hn R A
Mentha officinalis Hull, Brit. Fl. ed. 1, 127. 1799, incertae sedis. A

Menyanthes trifoliata L., Sp. Pl. 1: 145. 1753.
Menyanthaceae MENY. Hn R A F

Mercurialis perennis L., Sp. Pl. 2: 1035. 1753.
Euphorbiaceae MERL. Hn R G A

Mespilus laevigata see *Crataegus laevigata*

Metrosideros costata see *Angophora costata* subsp. *costata*

Mezereum see *Daphne mezereum*

Micromeria chamissonis Benth. in Greene, Man. Bot. San Francisco. 289. 1894.
Lamiaceae MICR. Hn R

Mikania amara Willd. var. **guaco** (Bonpl.) Baker, Fl. Bras. 6(2): 237. 1876.
Asteraceae GUA.
Mikania guaco Bonpl., Pl. Aequinoct. 2: 84, t. 105. 1809. Hs A
According to Index Kewensis *Mikania amara* Willd., (Comp. Rep.) is the accepted name of *Mikania guaco* Humb & Bonpl. Guaco (Hom. name) is the vernacular name.

Mikania guaco see *Mikania amara* var. *guaco*

Millefolium see *Achillea millefolium*

Mimosa dormiens Humb. & Bonpl. ex Willd., Willd., Sp. Pl. 4(2): 1035. 1806.
Fabaceae MIM-H. R
Mimosa humilis Humb. & Bonpl. ex Willd., Willd., Sp. Pl. 4(4): 1037. 1805. Hn A

Mimosa houstoniana see *Calliandra houstoniana*

Mimosa humilis see *Mimosa dormiens*

Mimosa pudica L., Sp. Pl. 1: 518. 1753.
Fabaceae MIM-P. Hn R

Mimosa quadrivalvis L. var. **angustata** (Torr. & A. Gray) Barneby, Mem. N.Y. Bot. Gard. 65. Sensitivae Censitae (Mimosa). 1991.
Fabaceae SCHRAN-U
Schrankia uncinata Willd., Willd., Sp. Pl 4(2): 1043. 1806. R

Mitchella repens L., Sp. Pl. 1: 111. 1753.
Rubiaceae MIT. Hn R A

Momordica balsamina L., Sp. Pl. 2: 1009. 1753.
Cucurbitaceae MOM-B. Hn R G A

Momordica charantia L., Sp. Pl. 2: 1009. 1753.
Cucurbitaceae MOM-CH. Hn R

Momordica elaterium see *Ecballium elaterium*

Momordica lanata see *Citrullus lanatus*

Annotated Checklist 61

Momordica operculata see *Luffa operculata*

➡ Monilia albicans see *Candida albicans*

Monsonia emarginata (L. f.) L'Hér., Geraniologia t. 41. 1792.
  Geraniaceae MONS.
  Geranium emarginatum L. f., Suppl. Pl. 306. 1782.
  Monsonia ovata Cav., Diss. 4: Quarta dissertatio botanica 193. 1787. Hn R
  The text for *Monsonia emarginata* (L. f.) L'herit., was not published until 1802.

Monsonia ovata see *Monsonia emarginata*

➡ **Mucor mucedo** L.: Fr., Sp. Pl. 2: 1185. 1753; Syst. Mycol. 3: 320. 1821.
  Mucoraceae MUCOR Hn R

Mucuna pruriens (L.) DC., Prodr. 2: 405. Nov 1825.
  Fabaceae DOL. R G A F
  Dolichos pruriens L., Herb. Amb. 23. 1754. Hn F
  Carpopogon pruriens (L.) Roxb., Hort. Bengal. 54. 1814. A

Mucuna urens (L.) Medik., Vorles. Churpfälz. Phys.-Öcon. Ges. 2: 399. 1787.

Fabaceae MUC-U. Hn R
  Dolichos urens L. Syst. Nat. ed. 10, 1162. 1759.

Musa paradisiaca var. sapientum see *Musa sapientum*

Musa sapientum L., Syst. Nat. ed. 10, 2: 1303. 1759.
  Musaceae MUSA Hn
  Musa paradisiaca L. var. *sapientum* (L.) Kuntze, Revis. Gen. Pl. 2: 692. 1891. R

Myosotis arvensis (L.) Hill, Veg. Syst. 7, ed. 1, 55. 1764.
  Boraginaceae MYOS-A. Hn R
  Myosotis scorpiodes L. var *arvensis* L., Sp. Pl. 1: 131. 1753.

Myosotis scorpiodes see *Myosotis arvensis*

Myrica cerifera L., Sp. Pl. 2: 1024. 1753.
  Myricaceae MYRIC. Hn R A

Myristica aromatica see *Myristica fragrans*

Myristica fragrans Houtt., Nat. Hist. 3: 333. 1775.
  Myristicaceae NUX-M. R G A F
  Myristica officinalis L. f., Suppl. Pl. 265. 1781. A
  Myristica moschata Thunb., Kongl. Vetensk. Acad. Nya Handl. 49. 1782. {Publication not seen} A
  Myristica aromatica Lam., Mém. Acad. Sci. (Paris) 1788: 155. 1791. A
  Linnaeus (1749 p. 179) uses Nux moschata as the medicinal name for *Myristica officinalis*.

Myristica moschata see *Myristica fragrans*

Myristica officinalis see *Myristica fragrans*

Myristica panamensis see *Myristica sebifera*

Myristica sebifera (Aubl.) Sw., Prodr. 96. 1788.
Myristicaceae MYRIS. Hn R
Virola sebifera Aubl., Hist. Pl. Guiane 2: 904, t. 345. 1775.
Myristica panamensis Hemsl., Biol. Cent.-Amer., Bot. 3: 67, t. 74. 1882. Hs

Myrospermum pereirae see *Myroxylon balsamum* var *pereirae*

Myrospermum toluiferum see *Myroxylon balsamum*

Myroxylon balsamum (L.) Harms, Notizbl. Konigl. Bot. Gart. Berlin 5: 94. 1908.
Fabaceae BALS-T.
Toluifera balsamum L., Sp. Pl. 1: 384. 1753.
Myroxylon toluiferum Kunth, Nov. Gen. Sp. 6: 375. 1824.
Myroxylon toluiferum A. Rich., Ann. Sci. Nat. (Paris) 2: 171. 1824. R
Myrospermum toluiferum (A. Rich.) DC., Prodr. 2: 95. Nov 1825.
Balsamum tolutanum [C. Bauhin] L., Pre-Linnaean name. Hn

Myroxylon balsamum (L.) Harms var. **pereirae** (Royle) Harms, Notizbl. Konigl. Bot. Gart. Berlin 43: 95. 1908.
Fabaceae BALS-P.
Myrospermum pereirae Royle, Man. Mat. Med. ed. 2, 414. 1853. A
Myroxylon pereirae Royle, Man. Mat. Med. ed. 2, 414. 1853. R
Royle in Man. Mat. Med. ed. 2, 414. 1853. indicates *Myrospermum pereirae* as Balsam of Peru.

Myroxylon pereirae see *Myroxylon balsamum* var. *pereirae*

Myroxylon toluiferum see *Myroxylon balsamum*

Myrtus cheken see *Luma chequen*

Myrtus chequen see *Luma chequen*

Myrtus communis L., Sp. Pl. 1: 471. 1753.
Myrtaceae MYRT-C. Hn R A

Myrtus cumini see *Syzygium cumini*

Myrtus dioica see *Pimenta dioica*

Myrtus jambos see *Syzygium jambos*

Nabalus serpentarius (Pursh) Hook., Fl. Bor.-Amer. 1: 294. 1840.
Asteraceae NABAL. Hn R A
Prenanthes serpentaria Pursh, Fl. Amer. Sept. 2: 499. 1814.

Narcissus poeticus L., Sp. Pl. 1: 289. 1753.
Amaryllidaceae NARC-PO. Hn R

Narcissus pseudonarcissus L., Sp. Pl. 1: 289. 1753.
Amaryllidaceae NARC-PS. Hn R

Narthex asafoetida see *Ferula narthex*

Nasturtium aquaticum see *Rorippa nasturtium-aquaticum*

Nasturtium officinale see *Rorippa nasturtium-aquaticum*

Nectandra amara Meisn., Prodr. 15(1): 158. Mai 1864.
Lauraceae NECT. Hn R

Nectandra coto see *Aniba coto*

Negundium see *Acer negundo*

Negundium americanum see *Acer negundo*

Nepenthes distillatoria L., Sp. Pl. 2: 955. 1753.
Nepenthaceae NEP. Hn R

Nepeta cataria L., Sp. Pl. 2: 570. 1753.
Lamiaceae NEPET. Hn R
Cataria nepeta abbreviated as CATAR (Comp. Rep., and Hom. name) is cited as a separate remedy and is an invalid combination.

Nepeta glechoma see *Glechoma hederacea*

Nepeta hederacea see *Glechoma hederacea*

Nerium oleander L., Sp. Pl. 1: 209. 1753.
Apocynaceae OLND. R Hs G A F
Common homeopathic name: Oleander.

Nicotiana tabacum L., Sp. Pl. 1: 180. 1753.
Solanaceae TAB. R Hs G A F
Linnaeus (1749 p. 29) uses Tabacum as the medicinal name for *Nicotiana tabacum*.

Nuphar lutea (L.) Sibth. & Sm., Fl. Graec. Prodr. I: 361. 1806.
Nymphaeaceae NUPH. Hn R A
Nymphaea lutea L., Sp. Pl. 1: 510. 1753. Hs A

Nux absurda see *Lodoicea maldivica*

Nux moschata see *Myristica fragrans*

Nux-vomica see *Strychnos nux-vomica*

Nyctanthes arbor-tristis L., Sp. Pl. 1: 6. 1753.
Oleaceae NYCT. Hn R

Nymphaea lutea see *Nuphar lutea*

Nymphaea odorata Aiton, Hort. Kew. 2: 227. 1789.
Nymphaeaceae NYM. Hn R A
Castalia pudica Salisb., Ann. Bot. (König & Sims) 2: 72. 1805. A

Ocimum canum Sims, Bot. Mag. 51: t. 2452. 1823.
Lamiaceae OCI. Hn R

Ocimum caryophyllatum Schweigg. ex Schrank, Denkschr. Königl.-Baier. Bot. Ges. Regensburg 2: 55. 1822.

Lamiaceae OCI-C. Hn R

Ocimum sanctum see *Ocimum tenuiflorum*

Ocimum tenuiflorum L., Sp. Pl. 2: 597. 1753.
Lamiaceae OCI-S.
Ocimum sanctum L., Mant. Pl. 1: 85. 1767. Hn R A

Odontonema rubrum (Vahl) Kuntze, Ann. Missouri Bot. Gard. 82(4): 542-548. 1995.
Acanthaceae JUST-R.
Justicia rubra Vahl, Eclog. Amer. 2: I. 1797.
Justicia "rubrum" (Comp. Rep.) is an orthographic variant.

Oenanthe aquatica (L.) Poir., Encycl. 4: 530. 1798.
Apiaceae PHEL. G F
Phellandrium aquaticum L., Sp. Pl. 1: 255. 1753. Hs A
Oenanthe phellandrium Lam., Fl. Franç. 3: 432. 1778. Hn R A F

Oenanthe crocata L., Sp. Pl. 1: 254. 1753.
Apiaceae OENA. Hn R A

Oenanthe phellandrium see *Oenanthe aquatica*

Oenothera biennis L., Sp. Pl. 1: 346. 1753.
Onagraceae OENO. Hn R A
Oenothera gauroides Hornem., Hort. Bot. Hafn. 1: 362. 1813, incertae sedis. A

Oenothera gauroides see *Oenothera biennis*

Oidium albicans see *Candida albicans*

Okoubaka aubrevillei Pellegr. & Normand, Bull. Soc. Bot. France 93: 139. 1946.
Santalaceae OKOU. Hn R

Oleander see *Nerium oleander*

Ononis spinosa L., Sp. Pl. 2: 716. 1753.
Fabaceae ONON. Hn R G

Onopordum acanthium L., Sp. Pl. 2: 827. 1753.
Asteraceae ONOP. Hn R

Onosmodium hispidium see *Onosmodium virginianum*

Onosmodium virginianum (L.) A. DC., Prodr. 10: 70. Apr 1846.
Boraginaceae ONOS. Hn R A
Lithospermum virginianum L., Sp. Pl. 1: 132. 1753. A
Onosmodium hispidum Michx., Fl. Bor.-Amer. ed. 1, 1: 133. 1803. A

Operculina turpethum (L.) Silva Manso, Enum. Subst. Braz. 16. 1836.
Convolvulaceae OPER. Hn
Convolvulus turpethum L., Sp. Pl. 1: 155. 1753.
Ipomoea turpethum (L.) R. Br., Prodr. ed. 1, 485. 1810. R

Ophioxylon serpentinum see *Rauwolfia serpentina*

Ophrys autumnalis see *Spiranthes spiralis*

Ophrys spiralis see *Spiranthes spiralis*

Opium see *Papaver somniferum*

Opuntia alba spina see *Opuntia microdasys*

Opuntia ficus-indica (L.) Mill., Gard. Dict. ed. 8. "Opuntia" 2. 1768.
Cactaceae OPUN-F. Hn R
Cactus ficus-indica L., Sp. Pl. 1: 468. 1753.

Opuntia microdasys (Lehm.) Pfeiff., Enum. Diagn. Cact. 154. 1837.
Cactaceae OPUN-A. R
Cactus microdasys Lehm., Sem. Hort. Bot. Hamburg 16. 1827.
Opuntia alba spina (Hom. name) is an unknown combination, the other nearest combination is the varietal name *Opuntia microdasys* var. *albispina* Fobe, Kakteenkunde 235. 1931.

Opuntia vulgaris Mill., Gard. Dict. ed. 8. "Opuntia" 1. 1768.
Cactaceae OPUN-V. Hn R A
Cactus opuntia L., Sp. Pl. 1: 468. 1753. A

Oreodaphne californica see *Umbellularia californica*

Origanum majorana L., Sp. Pl. 2: 590. 1753.
Lamiaceae ORIG. Hn R

Origanum vulgare L., Sp. Pl. 2: 590. 1753.
Lamiaceae ORIG-V. Hn R

Ornithogalum umbellatum L., Sp. Pl. 1: 307. 1753.
Hyacinthaceae ORNI. Hn R

Orobanche virginiana see *Epifagus virginiana*

Orthosiphon stamineus see *Clerodendranthus stamineus*

Osteospermum uvedalia see *Polymnia uvedalia*

Ostrya virginiana (Mill.) K. Koch, Dendrologie 2(2): 8. 1873.
Betulaceae OST. Hn R
Carpinus virginiana Mill., Gard. Dict. ed. 8. "Carpinus" 4. 1768.

Oxalis acetosella L., Sp. Pl. 1: 433. 1753.
Oxalidaceae OXAL. Hn R G

Oxydendrum arboreum (L.) DC., Prodr. 7(2): 601. Dec 1839.
Ericaceae OXYD. Hn R A
Andromeda arborea L., Sp. Pl. 1: 394. 1753.

Oxytropis lambertii Pursh, Fl. Amer. Sept. 2: 740. 1814.
Fabaceae OXYT. Hn R
Astragalus lambertii (Pursh) Spreng., Syst. Veg. 3: 308. 1826. R
Aragallus lambertii (Pursh) Greene, Pittonia 3: 212. 1897.

Astragalus lambertii abbreviated as ARAG. (Comp. Rep.) is cited as a separate remedy. *Aragallus "lamberti"*(Hom. name) is a typographic error.

Padus laurocerasus see *Prunus laurocerasus*

Paeonia officinalis L., Sp. Pl. 1: 530. 1753.
Ranunculaceae PAEON. Hn R G A F

Paloondo see *Larrea tridentata*

→ **Panaeolus papilionaceus** (Bull.: Fr.) Quél., Mém. Soc. Émul. Montbéliard. ser. 2, 5: 152. 1872.
Bolbitiaceae AGAR-CPN
Agaricus papilionaceus Bull.: Fr., Herb. France tome 2, pl. 58. 1781; Syst. Mycol. 1: 301. 1821.
Agaricus campanulatus Fr. (1753) Syst. Mycol. 1: 295. 1821, not L. 1753. Hn R
Agaricus campanulatus L., nom. dub., nom. excl., Sp. Pl. 2: 1175. 1753. This name is an excluded name as it is based on a different type and its identity obscure.

Panax pseudoginseng see *Aralia quinquefolia*

Panax quinquefolium see *Aralia quinquefolia*

Panax quinquefolius see *Aralia quinquefolia*

Panicum dactylon see *Cynodon dactylon*

Papaver somniferum L., Sp. Pl. 1: 508. 1753.
Papaveraceae OP. R A
Linnaeus (1749 p. 88) uses Opium as the medicinal name for *Papaver somniferum*.

Papaya vulgaris see *Carica papaya*

Pareira brava see *Chondrodendron tomentosum*

Parietaria officinalis L., Sp. Pl. 2: 1052. 1753.
Urticaceae PARIET. Hn R F

Paris quadrifolia L., Sp. Pl. 1: 367. 1753.
Trilliaceae PAR. Hn R G A

Parmelia pulmonacea see *Lobaria pulmonaria*

Paronychia illecebrum see *Alternanthera repens*

Parthenium hysterophorus L., Sp. Pl. 2: 988. 1753.
Asteraceae PARTH. Hn R

Parthenocissus quinquefolia (L.) Planch., Monogr. Phan. 5: 448. 1887.
Vitaceae AMPE-QU. R
Hedera quinquefolia L., Sp. Pl. 1: 202. 1753. A
Ampelopsis quinquefolia Michx., Fl. Bor.-Amer. ed. 1, 1: 160. 1803. Hn A

Passiflora incarnata L., Sp. Pl. 2: 959. 1753.

Passifloraceae PASSI. Hn R G A F

Pastinaca sativa L., Sp. Pl. 1: 262. 1753.
Apiaceae PAST. Hn R A

Paullinia cupana Kunth, Nov. Gen. Sp. 5: 117. 1821.
Sapindaceae PAULL. R A
Paullinia sorbilis Mart., Reise Bras. 1: 311. 1823. Hs A
Common homeopathic name: Guarana.

Paullinia pinnata L., Sp. Pl. 1: 366. 1753.
Sapindaceae PAULL-P. Hn R A
Incorrect usage: *Paullinia timbo* sensu Amer. Pharm., not Vell.

Paullinia sorbilis see *Paullinia cupana*

Paullinia timbo see *Paullinia pinnata*

Pelargonium reniforme Curtis, Bot. Mag. 14: t. 493. 1800.
Geraniaceae PELARG. Hn R

Pentaptera arjuna see *Terminalia arjuna*

Penthorum sedoides L., Sp. Pl. 1: 432. 1753.
Penthoraceae PEN. Hn R A

Periploca graeca L., Sp. Pl. 1: 211. 1753.
Asclepiadaceae PERI. Hn R

Periploca sylvestris see *Gymnema sylvestre*

Persea americana Mill., Gard. Dict. ed. 8. "Persea" 1. 1768.
Lauraceae PERS. Hn R G A
Persea gratissima C. F. Gaertn., Suppl. Carp. 3: 222, t. 221. 1807. G A

Persea gratissima see *Persea americana*

Petasites fragrans (Vill.) C. Presl, Fl. Sicul. 1: 28. 1826.
Asteraceae TUS-F. R
Tussilago fragrans Vill., Actes Soc. Hist. Nat. Paris 1: 72. 1792. Hn

Petasites hybridus (L.) P. Gaertn., B. Mey. & Scherb., Oekon. Fl. Wetterau 3: 184. 1801.
Asteraceae TUS-P.
Tussilago hybrida L., Sp. Pl. 2: 866. 1753.
Tussilago petasites L. Sp. Pl. 2: 866. 1753. Hn R

Petiveria alliacea L. var. **tetrandra** (Gomes) Hauman, Anales Mus. Nac. Hist. Nat. Buenos Aires 24: 501, 513. 1913.
Phytolaccaceae PETI.
Petiveria tetrandra Gomes, Mem. Math. Phis. Acad. Real Sci. Lisboa 3. 1812; Mem. Corresp. 17. {The date of publication could be 1814} Hn R

Petiveria tetrandra see *Petiveria alliacea* var. *tetranda*

Petroselinum see *Petroselinum crispum*

Petroselinum crispum (Mill.) Nyman ex A. W. Hill, Consp. Fl. Eur. 309. 1879. in obs.; Hand-list of Herbaceous Plants (Kew) ed. 3, 122. 1925.
Apiaceae PETROS. G
Apium crispum Mill., Gard. Dict. ed. 8. "Apium" 2. 1768.
Petroselinum sativum Hoffm., Gen. Pl. Umbell. 177. 1814. nom. nud. Hs A
Carum petroselinum (L.) Benth. & Hook. f., Gen. Pl. 1: 891. 1867. R A
Apium petroselinum L., Sp. Pl. 1: 264. 1753. Hs

Petroselinum sativum see *Petroselinum crispum*

Peucedanum oreoselinum (L.) Moench, Methodus 82. 1794.
Apiaceae ATHA. R
Athamanta oreoselinum L., Sp. Pl. 1: 244. 1753. A
"Athamantha" oreoselinum (Hom. name) is an orthographic variant.

Peucedanum ostruthium (L.) Koch, Nova Acta Phys.-Med. Acad. Caes. Leop.-Carol. Nat. Cur. 12(I): 95. 1824.
Apiaceae IMP. R
Imperatoria ostruthium L., Sp. Pl. 1: 259. 1753. Hn

Peumus boldus Molina, Sag. Stor. Nat. Chili 185, 350. 1782.
Monimiaceae BOLD. R G F
Boldea fragrans Gay, Fl. Chil. 5(3): 353. 1851 v. 1852.
"Boldo" fragrans (Hom. name) is an orthographic variant.

Phaca nuttallii see *Astragalus nuttallii*

Phalaris zizanioides see *Vetiveria zizanioides*

Phallus impudicus L.: Pers., Sp. Pl. 2: 1179. 1753; Syn. Meth. Fung., 242. 1801.
Phallaceae PHAL. Hn R

Phaseolus vulgaris L., Sp. Pl. 2: 723. 1753.
Fabaceae PHASE. Hn R

Phellandrium aquaticum see *Oenanthe aquatica*

Phleum pratense L., Sp. Pl. 1: 59. 1753.
Poaceae PHLE. Hn R

Phyla scaberrima (A. Juss. ex Pers.) Moldenke, Repert. Spec. Nov. Regni Veg., 41: 64. 1936.
Verbenaceae LIP.
Zapania scaberrima A. Juss. ex Pers., Syn. Pl. 2: 140. 1806.
Lippia mexicana Grieve, Modern Herb. 2: 831. 1931. Hn R A
Lippia dulcis Trevir., Nova Acta Phys.-Med. Acad. Caes. Leop.-Carol. Nat. Cur. 13(1): 187. 1826. A

Physalis alkekengi L., Sp. Pl. 1: 183. 1753.
Solanaceae PHYSAL. Hn R G

Physostigma venenosum Balf., Trans. Roy. Soc. Edinburgh 22: 310. 1861.
Fabaceae PHYS. Hn R A F

Phytolacca americana L., Sp. Pl. 1: 441. 1753.
    Phytolaccaceae **PHYT**. G A F
    Phytolacca decandra L., Sp. Pl. ed. 2, 2: 631. 1763. Hn R A F

Phytolacca decandra see *Phytolacca americana*

Picea mariana (Mill.) Britton, Sterns & Poggenb., Prelim. Cat. 71. 1888.
    Pinaceae **ABIES-N**. F
    Abies mariana Mill., Gard. Dict. ed. 8. "Abies" 5. 1768.
    Pinus nigra Aiton, Hort. Kew. 3: 370. 1789, not J.F. Arnold 1785. A
    Picea nigra (Aiton) Link, Handbuch 2: 478. 1831. Hs
    Abies nigra Du Roi, Harbk. Baumz. ed. 2, 182. 1800. Hn R A F
    Abies nigra (Aiton) Poir. Encycl. 6: 520. 1805.

Picea nigra see *Picea mariana*

Picrasma excelsa see *Quassia amara*

Pilocarpus jaborandi see *Pilocarpus microphyllus*

Pilocarpus microphyllus Stapf ex Wardleworth, Pharm. J. Trans. ser. 3, 24: 506. 1893. {Publication not seen}
    Rutaceae **JAB**. Hs G
    Pilocarpus microphyllus Stapf ex Holmes, Pharm. J. Trans. ser. 3, 24: 419. 1893, nom. inval. {Publication not seen}
    Pilocarpus microphyllus (1893) Stapf not Stapf ex Wardleworth, Bull. Misc. Inform. 4. 1894, nom. illeg. Hs G
    Jaborandi (Hom. name) is the name used for several pungent, aromatic, South American plants, notably *Pilocarpus* spp. Various species of *Pilocarpus* are used for the preparation of the remedy and these are mainly *Pilocarpus jaborandi* Holmes (Comp. Rep., and Germ. Pharm.), *Pilocarpus pennatifolius* Lem. (Amer. Pharm., Germ. Pharm., and Hom. syn.), and *Pilocarpus selloanus* Engl., (Amer. Pharm.).

Pilocarpus pennatifolius see *Pilocarpus microphyllus*

Pilocarpus selloanus see *Pilocarpus microphyllus*

Pimenta dioica (L.) Merr., Contr. Gray Herb. 165: 37, f. 1. 1947.
    Myrtaceae **PIME**.
    Myrtus dioica L., Syst. Nat. ed. 10, 1056. 1759.
    Pimenta officinalis Lindl., Coll. Bot. (4): pl. 19. 1821. Hn R

Pimenta officinalis see *Pimenta dioica*

Pimpinella alba see *Pimpinella saxifraga*

Pimpinella saxifraga L., Sp. Pl. 1: 263. 1753.
    Apiaceae **PIMP**. Hn R A
    Pimpinella alba Gueldenst., Reis. Russland 2: 192. 1791. {Publication not seen}. A

Pinus canadensis see *Tsuga canadensis*

Pinus excelsa see *Pinus lambertiana*

Pinus lambertiana Douglas, Trans. Linn. Soc. London 15: 500. 1827.
Pinaceae PIN-L. Hn R A
Incorrect usage: *Pinus excelsa* sensu Amer. Pharm., not D. Don.

Pinus nigra see *Picea mariana*

Pinus sylvestris L., Sp. Pl. 2: 1000. 1753.
Pinaceae PIN-S. Hn R G A F

Piper aduncum L., Sp. Pl. 1: 29. 1753.
Piperaceae MATI.
Piper angustifolium Lam., Tabl. Encycl. Tome 1: 81. 1791. R
Common homeopathic name: Matico.

Piper angustifolium see *Piper aduncum*

Piper cubeba L. f., Suppl. Pl. 90. 1782.
Piperaceae CUB. R A
Common homeopathic name: Cubeba.

Piper methysticum G. Forst., Pl. Esc. 76. 1786.
Piperaceae PIP-M. Hn R A
Macropiper methysticum Hook. & Arn. Bot. Beechey Voy. 96. 1832, incertae sedis, not Miq. 1843. A

Piper nigrum L., Sp. Pl. 1: 28. 1753.
Piperaceae PIP-N. Hn R A

Piscidia erythrina see *Piscidia piscipula*

Piscidia piscipula (L.) Sarg., Gard. & Forest 4: 436. 1891.
Fabaceae PISC.
Erythrina piscipula L., Sp. Pl. 2: 707. 1753.
Piscidia erythrina L., Syst. Nat. ed. 10, 2: 1155. 1759, nom. illeg. superfl. Hn R A

Plantago major L., Sp. Pl. 1: 112. 1753.
Plantaginaceae PLAN. Hn R F

Plantago minor Garsault, Fig. Pl. Méd. 3: t. 461. 1764.
Plantaginaceae PLAN-M. Hn R A

Platanus acerifolia see *Platanus x hispanica*

Platanus occidentalis see *Platanus x hispanica*

Platanus orientalis see *Platanus x hispanica*

Platanus x hispanica Mill. ex Münchh., Hausvater 5: 229. 1770.
Platanaceae PLATAN. G
Platanus x acerifolia (Aiton) Willd., Willd., Sp. Pl. 4(4): 474. 1805. R
Platanus orientalis L., Sp. Pl. 2: 999. 1753, pro parte.
Platanus occidentalis L., Sp. Pl. 2: 999. 1753, pro parte. G
Platanus occidentalis L. *Platanus x orientalis* L.

Platanus x acerifolia see *Platanus x hispanica*

Plectranthus amboinicus (Lour.) Spreng., Syst. Veg. 2: 690. 1825.
Lamiaceae COL-A.
Coleus amboinicus Lour., Fl. Cochinch. 2: 372. 1790.
Coleus aromaticus Benth., Pl. Asiat. Rar. 2: 15. 1831. Hn R

Plectranthus fruticosus L'Hér., Stirp. Nov. fasc. 4. 85. 1788.
Lamiaceae PLECT. Hn R A

Plumbago littoralis see *Plumbago scandens*

Plumbago scandens L., Sp. Pl. ed. 2, 1: 215. 1762.
Plumbaginaceae PLUMBG. R
Plumbago littoralis (Amer. Pharm., and Hom. name) is an unknown combination.

Podalyria tinctoria see *Baptisia tinctoria*

Podophyllum peltatum L., Sp. Pl. 1: 505. 1753.
Berberidaceae PODO. Hn R G A F

Polygala senega L., Sp. Pl. 2: 704. 1753.
Polygalaceae SENEG. R G A F
A mixture of *Polygala* spp. are used by the German and French pharmacopoeias. Common homeopathic name: Senega.

Polygonum acre see *Polygonum punctatum*

Polygonum aviculare L., Sp. Pl. 1: 362. 1753.
Polygonaceae POLYG-A. Hn R

Polygonum fagopyrum see *Fagopyrum esculentum*

Polygonum hydropiperoides see *Polygonum punctatum*

Polygonum persicaria L., Sp. Pl. 1: 361. 1753.
Polygonaceae POLYG-PE. Hn R

Polygonum punctatum Elliott, Sketch Bot. S. Carolina 1(5): 455. 1817.
Polygonaceae POLYG. Hs A
Polygonum hydropiperoides Pursh, Fl. Amer. Sept. 1: 270. 1814. Hn R A
Polygonum acre Kunth, Nov. Gen. Sp. 2: 179. 1817. Hs A

Polygonum sagittatum L., Sp. Pl. 1: 363. 1753.
Polygonaceae POLYG-S. Hn R

Polymnia uvedalia (L.) L., Sp. Pl. ed. 2, 2: 1303. 1763.
Asteraceae POLYM. Hn R
Osteospermum uvedalia L., Sp. Pl. 2: 923. 1753.

Polypodium filix-mas see *Dryopteris filix-mas*

Polyporus officinalis see *Fomitopsis officinalis*

Polyporus pinicola see *Fomitopsis pinicola*

Polyporus pinicolus see *Fomitopsis pinicola*

Polytrichum juniperinum Willd. ex Hedw., Sp. Musc. Frond 89, t. 18, fg. 6-10. 1801.
Polytrichaceae POLYTR. Hn R

Pontederia crassipes see *Eichhornia crassipes*

Populus balsamifera see *Populus x jackii*

Populus candicans see *Populus x jackii*

Populus gileadensis see *Populus x jackii*

Populus tremuloides Michx., Fl. Bor.-Amer. ed. 1, 2: 243. 1803.
Salicaceae POP. Hn R A

Populus x jackii Sarg., Trees & Shrubs 2: 212. 1913.
Salicaceae POP-C.
Populus gileadensis Rouleau, Rhodora 50: 235. 1948.
Populus candicans F. Michx. auct., not L. (1753) Hist. Arbr. Forest. 3: 308. 1813. Hn R
Populus balsamifera auct., (Hom. syn.) not L. (1753)

Potentilla anserina L., Sp. Pl. 1: 495. 1753.
Rosaceae POT-A. Hn R G

Potentilla erecta (L.) Raeusch., Nomencl. Bot. 152. 1797.
Rosaceae POT-T. R G
Tormentilla erecta L., Sp. Pl. 1: 500. 1753.
Potentilla tormentilla Neck., Hist. & Commentat. Acad. Elect. Sci. Theod.-Palat. 2: 491. 1770.
Potentilla "tomentilla"(Hom. name) is an orthographic variant.

Potentilla tomentilla see *Potentilla erecta*

Potentilla tormentilla see *Potentilla erecta*

Pothos foetidus see *Symplocarpus foetidus*

Prenanthes serpentaria see *Nabalus serpentarius*

Primula farinosa L., Sp. Pl. 1: 143. 1753.
Primulaceae PRIM-F. Hn R

Primula obconica Hance, J. Bot. 18(212): 234. 1880.
Primulaceae PRIM-O. Hn R

Primula veris L., Sp. Pl. 1: 142. 1753.
Primulaceae PRIM-V. Hn R

Prunus cerasifera Ehrh., Beitr. Naturk. 4: 17. 1789.
Rosaceae PRUN-C. Hn R

Prunus communis see *Prunus spinosa*

Prunus dulcis (Mill.) D. A. Webb, Feddes Repert. 74: 24. 1967.
Rosaceae AMYG-D. R
Amygdalus dulcis Mill., Gard. Dict. ed. 8. "Amygdalus" 2. 1768. Hn

Amygdalus communis L., Sp. Pl. 1: 473. 1753. Hs A
Amygdalus amara Hayne, Getreue Darstell. Gew. 4: 39, t. 39, f. 1. 1816. A
Prunus dulcis has a number of recognisable varieties that are still used in commerce: Bitter almond is *Prunus dulcis* var. *amara* (DC.) Focke (Germ. Pharm.), Sweet almond is *Prunus dulcis* var. *sativa* (Ludwig) Koch, and Brittle Almond is *Prunis dulcis* var *fragilis* (Borkh.) Focke.

Prunus laurocerasus L., Sp. Pl. 1: 474. 1753.
Rosaceae LAUR. R G A F
Padus laurocerasus Mill., Gard. Dict. ed. 8. "Padus" 4. 1768. A
Laurocerasus officinalis M. Roem., Fam. Nat. Syn. Monogr. 3 (Rosiflorae) 91. 1847. Hn

Prunus padus L., Sp. Pl. 1: 473. 1753.
Rosaceae PRUN-P. Hn R A

Prunus persica (L.) Batsch, Beytr. Entw. Gewächsreich 1: 30. 1801.
Rosaceae AMYG-P. R
Amygdalus persica L., Sp. Pl. 1: 472. 1753. Hn

Prunus serotina see *Prunus virginiana*

Prunus spinosa L., Sp. Pl. 1: 475. 1753.
Rosaceae PRUN. Hn R G A F
Prunus communis Huds., Fl. Angl. ed. 2, 1: 212. 1778, incertae sedis. A

Prunus virginiana L., Sp. Pl. 1: 473. 1753.
Rosaceae PRUN-V. Hn R A
Prunus serotina Poir., Encycl. 5: 665. 1804. A
Cerasus virginiana (L.) Michx., Fl. Bor.-Amer. ed. 1, 1: 285. 1803. Hs
Cerasus serotina Hook., Fl. Bor.-Amer. 1(4): 169. 1832, incertae sedis. A

Pseudotsuga menziesii (Mirb.) Franco, Bol. Soc. Brot., ser. 2, 24: 74. 1950.
Pinaceae PSEUTS-M. R

Psilocybe caerulescens Murrill, Mycologia 15: 20. 1923.
Strophariaceae PSIL. Hn R

Psoralea bituminosa L., Sp. Pl. 2: 763. 1753.
Fabaceae PSORAL. Hn R

Psychotria ipecacuanha (Brot.) Stokes, Bot. Mat. Med. 1: 365. 1812.
Rubiaceae IP.
Callicocca ipecacuanha Brot., Trans. Linn. Soc. London 6: 137. 1802. A
Cephaelis ipecacuanha (Brot.) A. Rich., Bull. Fac. Med. 4: 92. 1818. {Publication not seen} R G A F
Incorrect usage: *Cephaelis acuminata* sensu Fren. Pharm., not H. Karst. Common homeopathic name: Ipecacuanha. The French pharmacopoeia uses a mixture of species notably *Cephaelis acuminata* and *Cephaelis ipecacuanha*.

Ptelea trifoliata L., Sp. Pl. 1: 118. 1753.
Rutaceae PTEL. Hn R A F
Ptelea viticifolia Salisb., Prodr. Stirp. Chap. Allerton 68. 1796. A

Ptelea viticifolia see *Ptelea trifoliata*

Pulsatilla nigricans see *Pulsatilla pratensis*

Pulsatilla nuttalliana see *Pulsatilla patens*

Pulsatilla patens (L.) Mill., Gard. Dict. ed. 8. "Pulsatilla" 4. 1768.
  Ranunculaceae PULS-N.
  Anemone patens L., Sp. Pl. 1: 538. 1753. R A
  Pulsatilla nuttalliana Spreng., Syst. Veg. 2: 663. 1825. Hn
  Anemone nuttalliana DC., Syst. Nat. 1. 193. 1817, incertae sedis. A
  Anemone flavescens Zucc., Flora 9(1): 371. 1826, incertae sedis. A

Pulsatilla pratensis (L.) Mill., Gard. Dict. ed. 8. "Pulsatilla" 2. 1768.
  Ranunculaceae PULS. R G A
  Anemone pratensis L., Sp. Pl. 1: 539. 1753. Hs A
  Pulsatilla nigricans Störck, Libell. Pulsat. 7. 1771. Hn
  Incorrect usage: *Pulsatilla vulgaris* sensu Amer. and Fren. Pharm., not Mill.

Pulsatilla vulgaris see *Pulsatilla pratensis*

Punica granatum L., Sp. Pl. 1: 472. 1753.
  Lythraceae GRAN. R G A
  Common homeopathic name: Granatum.

Pyrethrum parthenium see *Tanacetum parthenium*

Pyrola corymbosa see *Chimaphila umbellata*

Pyrola maculata see *Chimaphila maculata*

Pyrola umbellata see *Chimaphila umbellata*

Pyrus americana (Marshall) DC., Prodr. 2: 637. Nov 1825.
  Rosaceae PYRUS Hn R A
  Sorbus americana Marshall, Arbust. Amer. 145. 1785.

Pyrus malus see *Malus pumila*

Quassia amara L., Sp. Pl. ed. 2, 1: 553. 1762.
  Simaroubaceae QUAS. Hn R G A
  Simaruba amara abbreviated as SIMA., is a separate remedy in the Complete repertory. Other species used for the preparation of the remedy are *Picrasma excelsa* (Sw.) Planch., (Germ. Pharm. and Hom. syn.) and *Quassia excelsa* Sw.

Quassia cedron see *Simaba cedron*

Quebracho see *Macaglia quebracho-blanco*

Quercus petraea see *Quercus robur*

Quercus robur L., Sp. Pl. 2: 996. 1753.
  Fagaceae QUERC-R. Hn R G
  Quercus robur var. *pedunculata* (Ehrh.) Hook.f. and *Quercus robur* var. *sessilifera* (Salisb.) Wahlb., (Hom. names) are varietal forms of *Quercus*

robur subsp. *robur* and *Quercus petraea* subsp.*petraea*. The German pharmacopoeia uses a mixture of *Quercus petraea* and *Quercus robur*.

Quillaja saponaria Molina, Sag. Stor. Nat. Chili 355. 1782.
Rosaceae QUILL. Hn R A

Radix Christopherianae see *Actaea spicata*

Rajania subsamarata see *Amphipterygium adstringens*

Ranunculus acris L., Sp. Pl. 1: 554. 1753.
Ranunculaceae RAN-A. Hn R A
Incorrect usage: *Ranunculus californicus* sensu Amer. Pharm., not Benth., *Ranunculus dissectus* sensu Amer. Pharm., not Hook. & Arn.

Ranunculus bulbosus L., Sp. Pl. 1: 554. 1753.
Ranunculaceae RAN-B. Hn R G A F

Ranunculus californicus see *Ranunculus acris*

Ranunculus dissectus see *Ranunculus acris*

Ranunculus flammula L., Sp. Pl. 1: 548. 1753.
Ranunculaceae RAN-FL. Hn R

Ranunculus glacialis L., Sp. Pl. 1: 553. 1753.
Ranunculaceae RAN-G. Hn R

Ranunculus palustris see *Ranunculus sceleratus*

Ranunculus repens L., Sp. Pl. 1: 554. 1753.
Ranunculaceae RAN-R. Hn R A

Ranunculus sceleratus L., Sp. Pl. 1: 551. 1753.
Ranunculaceae RAN-S. Hn R A
Ranunculus palustris Garsault, Fig. Pl. Méd. 4: t. 485. 1764, incertae sedis. A

Raphanus niger see *Raphanus sativus*

Raphanus nigrum see *Raphanus sativus*

Raphanus sativus L., Sp. Pl. 2: 669. 1753.
Brassicaceae RAPH. Hn R A
Raphanus nigrum Mill., Gard. Dict. ed. 8. "Raphanus" 4. 1768. A
Raphanus nigrum has been sunk into *R. sativus* (*Raphanus sativus* var *niger*, Germ., and Fren. Pharm.). The variety seems to be little different from the type. *Raphanus "niger"* (Fren. Pharm.) is an orthographic variant.

Ratanhia peruviana see *Krameria lappacea*

Rauvolfia serpentina see *Rauwolfia serpentina*

Rauwolfia serpentina (L.) Benth. ex Kurz, Forest. Fl. Burma 2: 171. 1878.
Apocynaceae RAUW. Hn G A
Ophioxylon serpentinum L., Sp. Pl. 2: 1043. 1753.
"Rauvolfia" serpentina (Comp. Rep.) is an orthographic variant of *Rauwolfia*

serpentina.

Rhamnus californica Eschsch., Mém. Acad. St.-Pétersb. 10: 285. 1823.
Rhamnaceae **RHAM-CAL** Hn R

Rhamnus cathartica L., Sp. Pl. 1: 193. 1753.
Rhamnaceae **RHAM-CAT** Hn R A H.
Incorrect usage: *Frangula caroliniana* sensu Amer. Pharm., not A. Gray.

Rhamnus frangula see *Frangula alnus*

Rhamnus humboldtiana see *Karwinskia humboldtiana*

Rhamnus purshiana DC. Prodr. 2: 25. Nov 1825, "purshianus".
Rhamnaceae **RHAM-P**. R Hs A
Cascara sagrada (Amer. Pharm., and Hom. name) is the vernacular name.

Rheum compactum see *Rheum palmatum*

Rheum emodi see *Rheum palmatum*

Rheum officinale see *Rheum palmatum*

Rheum palmatum L., Syst. Nat. ed. 10, 2: 1010. 1759.
Polygonaceae **RHEUM** Hn R G A F
Incorrect usage: *Rheum compactum* sensu Amer. Pharm., not L., and *Rheum emodi* sensu Amer. Pharm., not Wall. The French and German pharmacopoeias use a mixture of *Rheum palmatum* L. and *Rheum officinale* Baill.

Rhododendron aureum Georgi, Reise Russ. Reich. 1: 51, 214. 1775.
Ericaceae **RHOD**. R
Rhododendron officinale Salisb., Parad. Lond. t. 80. 1807. A
Rhododendron chrysanthum Pall., Reise Russ. Reich. 3(2): 729. 1776. Hn
Incorrect usage: *Rhododendron campylocarpum* sensu Germ. Pharm., not Hook. f. and *Rhododendron ferrugineum* sensu Fren. Pharm., not L.
Rhododendron chrysanth(em)um sic. (Amer. Pharm.).

Rhododendron campylocarpum see *Rhododendron aureum*

Rhododendron chrysanthemum see *Rhododendron aureum*

Rhododendron chrysanthum see *Rhododendron aureum*

Rhododendron ferrugineum see *Rhododendron aureum*

Rhododendron officinale see *Rhododendron aureum*

Rhus aromatica Aiton, Hort. Kew. 1: 367. 1789.
Anacardiaceae **RHUS-A**. Hn R A
Rhus suaveolens Aiton, Hort. Kew. 1: 368. 1789. Hs A
Rhus canadense Marshall, Arbust. Amer. 129. 1785, not Mill. 1768.
Rhus "canadensis" (Amer. Pharm., and Hom. syn.) is an orthographic variant.

Rhus canadense see *Rhus aromatica*

Rhus canadensis see *Rhus aromatica*

Rhus carolinense see *Rhus glabra*

Rhus diversiloba see *Toxicodendron diversilobum*

Rhus elegans see *Rhus glabra*

Rhus glabra L., Sp. Pl. 1: 265. 1753.
Anacardiaceae RHUS-G. Hn R A
Rhus glabra var. *elegans* (Aiton) Engl., Monogr. Phan. 4: 377. 1882.
Rhus elegans Aiton, Hort. Kew. 1: 366. 1789. Hs A
Rhus carolinense Marshall, Arbust. Amer. 129. 1785, incertae sedis. Hs A

Rhus laurina see *Malosma laurina*

Rhus radicans see *Toxicodendron radicans*

Rhus suaveolens see *Rhus aromatica*

Rhus toxicodendron see *Toxicodendron pubescens*

Rhus venenata see *Toxicodendron vernix*

Rhus vernix see *Toxicodendron vernix*

Rhus verrucosa see *Toxicodendron pubescens*

Ricinus africanus see *Ricinus communis*

Ricinus communis L., Sp. Pl. 2: 1007. 1753.
Euphorbiaceae RIC. Hn R A F
Ricinus viridis Willd., Willd., Sp. Pl. 4(1): 564. 1805. A
Ricinus africanus Mill., Gard. Dict. ed. 8. "Ricinus" 5. 1768. A

Ricinus viridis see *Ricinus communis*

Robinia fragilis see *Robinia pseudoacacia*

Robinia pseudoacacia L., Sp. Pl. 2: 722. 1753.
Fabaceae ROB. Hn R A F
Robinia fragilis Salisb., Prodr. Stirp. Chap. Allerton 336. 1796. A

Rorella rotundifolia see *Drosera rotundifolia*

Rorippa nasturtium-aquaticum (L.) Hayek, Sched. Fl. Stiriac. 3-4: 22. 1905.
Brassicaceae NAST.
Sisymbrium nasturtium-aquaticum L., Sp. Pl. 2: 657. 1753.
Nasturtium officinale R. Br., Hortus Kew. 4: 110. 1812. G
Nasturtium aquaticum Garsault, Fig. Pl. Méd. 3: t. 403. 1764. Hn R

Rosa damascena Mill., Gard. Dict. ed. 8. "Rosa" 15. 1768.
Rosaceae ROS-D. Hn R

Rosmarinus officinalis L., Sp. Pl. 1: 23. 1753.
Lamiaceae ROSM. Hn R G F

Rottlera tinctoria see *Mallotus philippensis*

Rubia tinctorum L., Sp. Pl. 1: 109. 1753.

Rubiaceae RUB-T. Hn R

Rudbeckia angustifolia see *Echinacea angustifolia*

Rudbeckia pallida see *Echinacea angustifolia*

Rudbeckia purpurea see *Echinacea purpurea*

Rumex acetosa L., Sp. Pl. 1: 337. 1753.
Polygonaceae RUMX-A. Hn R A

Rumex crispus L., Sp. Pl. 1: 335. 1753.
Polygonaceae RUMX. Hn R G A F

Rumex obtusifolius L., Sp. Pl. 1: 335. 1753.
Polygonaceae LAPA. R
Lapathum (Hom. name) is the vernacular name

Russula emetica (Schaeff.: Fr) Gray, Nat. Arr. Brit. Pl. 1: 618. 1821.
Russulaceae AGAR-EM. R A
Agaricus emeticus Schaeff.: Fr., Fung. Bavar. Palat. Nasc. 1: 9. t. 15. 1762; Syst. Mycol. 1: 56. 1821. Hn A

Russula foetens Pers.: Fr., Syn. Meth. Fung. 2: 443. 1801; Syst. Mycol. 1: 59. 1821.
Russulaceae RUSS. Hn R

Ruta graveolens L., Sp. Pl. 1: 383. 1753.
Rutaceae RUTA Hn R G A F
Ruta hortensis Mill., Gard. Dict. ed. 8. "Ruta" 1. 1768. A

Ruta hortensis see *Ruta graveolens*

Sabadilla officinalis see *Schoenocaulon officinale*

Sabal serrulata see *Serenoa repens*

Sabal serrulatum see *Serenoa repens*

Sabina see *Juniperus sabina*

Sabina officinalis see *Juniperus sabina*

Saccharomyces cerevisiae Meyen ex E. C. Hansen, Arch. Naturgesch. 4(2): 100. 1838.
Saccharomycetaceae TORUL.
Torula cerevisiae Turpin, Compt. Rend. 7(8): 379. 1838. Hn R

Saccharum officinarum L., Sp. Pl. 1: 54. 1753.
Poaceae SAC-ALB. Hn R

Salix amygdalina see *Salix triandra*

Salix falcata see *Salix nigra*

Salix helix see *Salix purpurea*

Salix mollissima Hoffm. ex Elwert, Fasc. Pl. Fl. Marggrav. 21. 1786.

Salicaceae SALX-M. Hn R

Salix monandra see *Salix purpurea*

Salix nigra Marshall, Arbust. Amer. 293. 1785.
Salicaceae SALX-N. Hn R A
Salix falcata Pursh, Fl. Amer. Sept. 2: 614. 1814. A
Salix purshiana Spreng., Syst. Veg. 5 (Index): 608. 1828. A

Salix purpurea L., Sp. Pl. 2: 1017. 1753.
Salicaceae SALX-P. Hn R A
Salix monandra Hoffm., Hist. Salic. ill. 1(1): 18. 1785.
Salix monandra Ard. Mem. Osserv. Var. Piante 1: 67, t. 11. 1766, incertae sedis. A
Salix helix L., Sp. Pl. 2: 1017. 1753, incertae sedis. A

Salix purshiana see *Salix nigra*

Salix triandra L., Sp. Pl. 2: 1016. 1753.
Salicaceae SALX-AM.
Salix amygdalina L., Sp. Pl. 2: 1016. 1753. Hn R

Salvia officinalis L., Sp. Pl. 1: 23. 1753.
Lamiaceae SALV. Hn R G A F

Salvia sclarea L., Sp. Pl. 1: 27. 1753.
Lamiaceae SALV-SC. Hn R

Sambucus canadensis L., Sp. Pl. 1: 269. 1753.
Caprifoliaceae SAMB-C. Hn R A
Sambucus humilis Raf., Ann. Nat. 13. 1820, not Mill. 1768. Hs A
Sambucus glauca Nutt. ex Torr. & Gray, Fl. N. Amer. 2: 13. 1841, cited that this species is hardly distinguishable from *S. canadensis*. Hs A

Sambucus glauca see *Sambucus canadensis*

Sambucus humilis see *Sambucus canadensis*

Sambucus nigra L., Sp. Pl. 1: 269. 1753.
Caprifoliaceae SAMB. Hn R G A F

Samyda guidonia see *Guarea guidonia*

Sanguinaria canadensis L., Sp. Pl. 1: 505. 1753.
Papaveraceae SANG. Hn R G A F
Sanguinaria vernalis Salisb., Prodr. Stirp. Chap. Allerton 376. 1796. A
Sanguinaria grandiflora M. Roscoe, Fl. Ill. Seasons, t. 8; 1829. A

Sanguinaria grandiflora see *Sanguinaria canadensis*

Sanguinaria vernalis see *Sanguinaria canadensis*

Sanguisorba officinalis L., Sp. Pl. 1: 116. 1753.
Rosaceae SANGUIS. Hn R

Santalum album L., Sp. Pl. 1: 349. 1753.

Santalaceae SANTA. Hn R

Saponaria officinalis L., Sp. Pl. 1: 408. 1753.
Caryophyllaceae SAPO. Hn R F

Saraca asoca (Roxb.) De Wild., Blumea 15: 393. 1968.
Fabaceae JOAN.
Jonesia asoca Roxb., Asiat. Res. 4: 355. 1795.
"*Joanesia*" *asoca* (Comp. Rep.) is a typographic error. *Saraca indica* L. is a valid name but the plant used in homeopathy is *Jonesia asoca*. "The common Saraca (Indian Sorrowless Tree) was almost always refered to *Saraca indica* L. It appeared, however, that the type specimen of *Saraca indica* L., collected from Java belongs to a different species. The species occurring in Ceylon, India, Bangla Desh and Burma, west of the Irrawaddy River has been determined as *Saraca asoca* (Roxb.) De Wilde, based on *Jonesia asoca* Roxb." (Manilal 1980, p.221).

Saraca indica see *Saraca asoca*

Sarothamnus scoparius see *Cytisus scoparius*

Sarracenia gronovii see *Sarracenia purpurea*

Sarracenia purpurea L., Sp. Pl. 1: 510. 1753.
Sarraceniaceae SARR. Hn R A
Incorrect usage: *Sarracenia gronovii* sensu Amer. Pharm., not A. W. Wood.

Sarsaparilla officinalis see *Smilax regelii*

Satureja hortensis L., Sp. Pl. 2: 568. 1753.
Lamiaceae SAT. Hn R

Scammonium see *Convolvulus scammonia*

Schinus molle L., Sp. Pl. 1: 388. 1753.
Anacardiaceae SCHIN. Hn R

Schoenocaulon officinale (Schltdl. & Cham.) A. Gray ex Benth. Pl. Hartw. 29. 1840.
Melanthiaceae SABAD. R G A
Veratrum officinale Schltdl. & Cham., Linnaea 6: 45. 1831. Hs
Sabadilla officinalis (Schltdl. & Cham.) Standl., Lista Pl. Salvador. 49. 1925. Hn
Asagraea officinalis (Schltdl. & Cham.) Lindl., Sketch Veg. Swan R. 25: 33. 1839. {Publication not seen} Hs

Schrankia uncinata see *Mimosa quadrivalvis* var. *angustata*

Scilla alba see *Drimia maritima*

Scilla maritima see *Drimia maritima*

Scilla nutans see *Hyacinthoides non-scripta*

Scleranthus annuus L., Sp. Pl. 1: 406. 1753.
Illecebraceae SCLER-A. Hn R

Scolopendrium vulgare see *Asplenium scolopendrium*

Scopolia carniolica Jacq., Observ. Bot. 1: 32. 1764.
Solanaceae SCOPO. Hn R

Scrophularia foetida see *Scrophularia nodosa*

Scrophularia nodosa L., Sp. Pl. 2: 619. 1753.
Scrophulariaceae SCROPH-N. Hn R G A F
Scrophularia foetida Garsault, Fig. Pl. Méd. 4: t. 533. 1764. A

Scutellaria lateriflora L., Sp. Pl. 2: 598. 1753.
Lamiaceae SCUT. Hn
Scutellaria "laterifolia" (Comp. Rep., and Amer. Pharm.) is an unknown combination. The nearest combination is *Scutellaria lateriflora,* which is also the species used in the proving by Hale.

Scutellaria laterifolia see *Scutellaria lateriflora*

⟶ Secale cornutum see *Claviceps purpurea*

Sedum acre L., Sp. Pl. 1: 432. 1753.
Crassulaceae SED-AC. Hn R

Sedum alpestre Vill., Prosp. Hist. Pl. Dauphiné. 49. 1779.
Crassulaceae SED-R.
Sedum repens Schleich. ex DC., Fl. Franç. ed. 3, 5: 525. 1815. Hn R

Sedum repens see *Sedum alpestre*

Sedum telephium see *Hylotelephium telephium*

Selenicereus grandiflorus (L.) Britton & Rose, Contr. U. S. Natl. Herb. 12: 430. 1909.
Cactaceae CACT. R G A F
Cactus grandiflorus L., Sp. Pl. 1: 467. 1753. Hn
Cereus grandiflorus Mill., Gard. Dict. ed. 8. "Cereus" 11. 1768. A F

Semecarpus anacardium L. f., Suppl. Pl. 182. 1782.
Anacardiaceae ANAC. R G F
Anacardium officinarum Gaertn., Fruct. Sem. Pl. 1(1): 192. 1788. Hs
Linnaeus (1749 p. 14) uses Anacardium orientale (Hom. name) as the medicinal name.

Sempervivum tectorum L., Sp. Pl. 1: 464. 1753.
Crassulaceae SEMP. Hn R G A
Sempervivum tectorum L. subsp. *tectorum* (Germ. Pharm.) is the same as *Sempervivum tectorum.*

Senecio aureus L., Sp. Pl. 2: 870. 1753.
Asteraceae SENEC. Hn R A
Incorrect usage: *Senecio gracilis (*Amer. Pharm., and Hom. syn.), not Pursh.

Senecio bicolor (Willd.) Tod. subsp. **cineraria** (DC.) Chater, Bot. J. Linn. Soc. 68: 273. 1974.
Asteraceae CINE. F

Senecio cineraria DC., Prodr. 6: 355. Jan 1838. Hs A
Senecio maritimus Rchb. Mössler's Handb. Gewächsk. ed. 2, 2: 1479. 1834, not L. f. 1782. F
Cineraria maritima L., Sp. Pl. ed. 2, 2: 925. 1763. Hn R A

Senecio cineraria see *Senecio bicolor* subsp. *cineraria*

Senecio gracilis see *Senecio aureus*

Senecio hieracifolius see *Erechtites hieracifolia*

Senecio hieraciifolius see *Erechtites hieracifolia*

Senecio jacobaea L., Sp. Pl. 2: 870. 1753.
Asteraceae SENEC-J. Hn R

Senecio maritimus see *Senecio bicolor* subsp. *cineraria*

Senega   see *Polygala senega*

Senna   see *Senna alexandrina*

Senna alexandrina Mill., Gard. Dict. ed. 8. "Senna" 1. 1768.
Fabaceae SENN. Hs
Cassia senna L., Sp. Pl. 1: 377. 1753. A F
Cassia angustifolia Vahl, Symb. Bot. 1: 29. 1790. F
Cassia acutifolia Delile, Descr. Égypte, Hist. Nat. 61, t. 27. 1813. R A F
Several species of *Cassia* are cited for the preparation of Senna (Hom.name). The species used mainly are *Senna alexandriana* Mill., and *Cassia obovata* Collad.

Senna sophera (L.) Roxb., Fl. Ind. ed. 1832. 2: 347. 1832.
Fabaceae CASSI-S.
Cassia sophera L., Sp. Pl. 1: 379. 1753. Hn

Sequoia sempervirens (D. Don) Endl., Syn. Conif. 198. 1847.
Taxodiaceae SEQ-S. Hn R
Taxodium sempervirens D. Don, Descr. Pinus 2: 24. 1824.

Serenoa repens (W. Bartram) Small, J. New York Bot. Gard. 27(321): 197. 1926.
Arecaceae SABAL. G
Corypha repens W. Bartram, Travels Carolina 61. 1791.
Serenoa serrulata Hook.f. in Benth. & Hook., Gen. Pl. 3(2): 926. 1883. Hs
Sabal serrulata (Michx.) Nutt. ex Schult. & Schult.f., Syst. Veg. 7: 1486. 1830. Hn R A
Brahea serrulata (Michx.) H. Wendl., Bot Zeitung (Berlin) 37: 147. 1879. F

Serenoa serrulata see *Serenoa repens*

Seriphidium maritimum (L.) Poljakov, Trudy Inst. Bot. Akad. Nauk Kazakhst. S S R, 11:172. 1961.
Asteraceae CINA
Artemisia maritima L., Sp. Pl. 2: 846. 1753. R A
Artemisia contra Willd. ex Spreng, Syst. Veg. 3: 494. 1826,

not L. 1753. Hs A
Incorrect usage: *Artemisia cina* sensu Fren. Pharm., not Berg ex Poljakov.
Common homeopathic name: Cina.

Serpentaria virginiana see *Aristolochia serpentaria*

Serratula spicata see *Liatris spicata*

Sigesbeckia orientalis L., Sp. Pl. 2: 900. 1753.
Asteraceae SIEG. Hn R

Silphium laciniatum L., Sp. Pl. 2: 919. 1753.
Asteraceae SILPHU. Hn R A

Silybum marianum (L.) Gaertn., Fruct. Sem. Pl. 2(3): 378, t. 162. 1791.
Asteraceae CARD-M. R G A F
Carduus marianus L., Sp. Pl. 2: 823. 1753. Hn A

Simaba cedron Planch., London J. Bot. 5: 566. 1846.
Simaroubaceae CEDR. Hs A F
Quassia cedron Baill., Hist. Pl. 4: 406. 1873. F
Incorrect usage: The generic name "*Simaruba*" as in *Simaruba cedron* (Germ. and Amer. Pharm.) and *Simaruba ferruginea* (Comp. Rep.) is rejected. The current accepted generic name is "*Simaba*". *Simaba ferruginea* sensu Comp. Rep., not A. St.-Hil. Common homeopathic name: Cedron.

Simaba ferruginea see *Simaba cedron*

Simarouba amara Aubl., Hist. Pl. Guiane 2:860, t. 331-332. 1775.
Simaroubaceae SIMA. R

Simaruba cedron see *Simaba cedron*

Simaruba ferroginea see *Simaba cedron*

Sinapis alba see *Brassica alba*

Sinapis nigra see *Brassica nigra*

Sisymbrium nasturtium-aquaticum see *Rorippa nasturtium-aquaticum*

Sisyrinchium galaxioides see *Trimezia galaxioides*

Sisyrinchium galaxoides see *Trimezia galaxioides*

Sium latifolium L., Sp. Pl. 1: 251. 1753.
Apiaceae SIUM Hn R

Smilax aristolochiifolia see *Smilax regelii*

Smilax medica see *Smilax regelii*

Smilax officinalis see *Smilax regelii*

Smilax regelii Killip & C. V. Morton, Publ. Carnegie Inst. Wash. 461(12): 272. 1936.
Smilacaceae SARS.
Smilax sarsaparilla L., Sp. Pl. 2: 1029. 1753. Hs A

Smilax officinalis Kunth, Nov. Gen. Sp. 1: 271. 1816. A
Incorrect usage: *Smilax aristolochiifolia* sensu Fren. Pharm., not Mill., and *Smilax medica* sensu Amer., and Fren. Pharm., not Schlecht & Cham. *Sarsaparilla officinalis* (Comp. Rep., and Hom. name) is an invalid name. Different species of *Smilax* are used by the American and French Pharmacopoeias.

Smilax sarsaparilla see *Smilax regelii*

Smyrnium aureum see *Zizia aurea*

Solanum aethiopicum L., Cent. Pl. 2, 10. 1756.
Solanaceae SOL-I.
Solanum integrifolium Poir., Encycl. 4: 301. 1797.
Solanum "integri" (Comp. Rep.) is a typographic error.

Solanum americanum Mill., Gard. Dict. ed. 8. "Solanum" 5. 1768.
Solanaceae SOL-O.
Solanum oleraceum Dunal ex Poir., Encycl. Suppl. 3: 750. 1814. Hn R

Solanum arrebenta see *Solanum capsicoides*

Solanum capsicoides All., Mélanges Philos. Math. Soc. Roy. Turin 5: 64. 1773.
Solanaceae SOL-A. R
Solanum ciliatum Lam., Tabl. Encycl. Tome 2: 21. 1794, pro parte.
Solanum arrebenta Vell., Fl. Flumin. 89. 1829; Icones 2: [i], pl. 127. 1827.
Also see Taxon 22: 281. 1973. Hn A

Solanum carolinense L., Sp. Pl. 1: 187. 1753.
Solanaceae SOL-C. Hn R A

Solanum ciliatum see *Solanum capsicoides*

Solanum dulcamara L., Sp. Pl. 1: 185. 1753.
Solanaceae DULC. R G A F

Solanum integri see *Solanum aethiopicum*

Solanum integrifolium see *Solanum aethiopicum*

Solanum lycopersicum L., Sp. Pl. 1: 185. 1753.
Solanaceae LYCPR. Hs.A
Lycopersicon lycopersicum (L.) H. Karst., Deut. Fl. ed. 1. lief. 966. 1882, nom. rejic.
Lycopersicon esculentum Mill., Gard. Dict. ed. 8. "Lycopersicon" 1. 1768. Hn R A

Solanum mammosum L., Sp. Pl. 1: 187. 1753.
Solanaceae SOL-M. Hn R A

Solanum nigrum L., Sp. Pl. 1: 186. 1753.
Solanaceae SOL-N. Hn R A

Solanum oleraceum see *Solanum americanum*

Solanum pseudocapsicum L., Sp. Pl. 1: 184. 1753.
Solanaceae SOL-PS. Hn R

Solanum tuberosum L., Sp. Pl. 1: 185. 1753.
Solanaceae SOL-T. Hn R

Solanum virginianum L., Sp. Pl. 1: 187. 1753.
Solanaceae SOL-X.
Solanum xanthocarpum Schrad. & H. Wendl., Sert. Hannov. 1: 8. pl. 2. 1795.
Solanum "xanthocarpus" (Comp. Rep.) is an orthographic variant.

Solanum xanthocarpum see *Solanum virginianum*

Solanum xanthocarpus see *Solanum virginianum*

Solidago virga aurea see *Solidago virgaurea*

Solidago virgaurea L., Sp. Pl. 2: 880. 1753.
Asteraceae SOLID. Hn R G A
Solidago "virga aurea" (Fren. Pharm.) appears to be a typographic error.

Sophora australis see *Baptisia australis*

Sophora tinctoria see *Baptisia tinctoria*

Sorbus americana see *Pyrus americana*

Spartium scoparium see *Cytisus scoparius*

→ Sphaeria purpurea see *Claviceps purpurea*

Spigelia anthelmia L., Sp. Pl. 1: 149. 1753.
Loganiaceae SPIG. Hn R G A F

Spigelia marilandica (L.) L., Syst. Nat. ed. 12, 734. 1767.
Loganiaceae SPIG-M. Hn R
Lonicera marilandica L., Syst. Nat. ed. 12, 166. 1767.

Spiraea ulmaria see *Filipendula ulmaria*

Spiranthes autumnalis see *Spiranthes spiralis*

Spiranthes spiralis (L.) Chevall., Fl. Gén. Env. Paris 2: 330. 1827.
Orchidaceae SPIRA.
Ophrys spiralis L., Sp. Pl. 2: 945. 1753.
Spiranthes autumnalis (Balb.) Rich., De Orchid. Eur. 37. 1817, nom. illeg. superfl. Hn R
Ophrys autumnalis Balb., Elench. Pl. Nov. 96. 1801.

Squill see *Drimia maritima*

Stachys betonica see *Stachys officinalis*

Stachys officinalis (L.) Trevis., Das Natürliche Pflanzensystem, 4, 3a: 216. 1897.
Lamiaceae STACH. R G
Betonica officinalis L., Sp. Pl. 2: 573. 1753.

Stachys betonica Benth., Labiat. Gen. Spec. 532. 1834. Hn

Staphysagria see *Delphinium staphisagria*

Stellaria media (L.) Vill., Hist. Pl. Dauphiné 3(2): 615. 1789.
Caryophyllaceae STEL. Hn R
Alsine media L., Sp. Pl. 1: 272. 1753.

Sterculia acuminata see *Cola acuminata*

Sticta pulmonacea see *Lobaria pulmonaria*

Sticta pulmonaceae see *Lobaria pulmonaria*

Sticta pulmonaria see *Lobaria pulmonaria*

Stigmata maydis see *Zea mays*

Stillingia sylvatica L., Mant. Pl. 1: 126. 1767.
Euphorbiaceae STILL. Hn R A

Stramonium see *Datura stramonium*

Stramonium foetidum see *Datura stramonium*

Strophanthus gratus see *Strophanthus kombe*

Strophanthus hispidus var. kombe see *Strophanthus kombe*

Strophanthus kombe Oliv., Icon. Pl. 79, t. 1098. 1871.
Apocynaceae STROPH. A
Strophanthus hispidus var. *kombe* (Oliv.) Holmes, Belmontia, n.s. 13: 96. 1982.
Incorrect usage: *Strophanthus gratus* sensu Germ. Pharm., not (Wall. et Hook.) Franch.
Strophanthus hispidus DC (Hom.name, Comp. Rep., and Amer. Pharm.) is also used for the preparation of the remedy.

Strophanthus sarmentosus DC., Bull. Sci. Soc. Philom. Paris 3: 123, t. 8, f. 1. 1802.
Apocynaceae STROPH-S. Hn R A

Stropharia semiglobata (Batsch: Fr.) Quél., Champ. Jura Vosges 1: 112. 1872.
Strophariaceae AGAR-SE.
Agaricus semiglobatus Batsch.: Fr., Elench. Fung. f. 110. 1783; Syst. Mycol. 1: 284. 1821. Hn R

Strychnos axillaris Colebr., Trans. Linn. Soc. London 12(2): 356, t. 15. 1818.
Loganiaceae HO.
Strychnos malaccensis Pierre ex C. B. Clarke, Fl. Brit. India 4(10): 89. 1883. Hs
Strychnos gauthierana Pierre ex Dop, Bull. Soc. Bot. France 57(19): 17. 1909.
Strychnos "*gaulthierana*" (Comp. Rep.) is a typographic error. Hoang-nan (Hom. name) is the vernacular name.

Strychnos gaultheriana see *Strychnos axillaris*

Strychnos gauthierana see *Strychnos axillaris*

Strychnos ignatii P. J. Bergius, Mater. Med. 1: 146. 1778.
Loganiaceae IGN. R G A F
Ignatia amara L. f., Suppl. Pl. 149. 1782. Hn F

Strychnos malaccensis see *Strychnos axillaris*

Strychnos nux-vomica L., Sp. Pl. 1: 189. 1753.
Loganiaceae NUX-V. R G A F
Linnaeus (1749 p. 26) uses Nux vomica as the medicinal name for *Strychnos nux-vomica*.

Strychnos tieute Lesch., Ann. Mus. Par. 16: 479, 480. t. 23. 1810.
Loganiaceae UPA. R
The name Upas tieute (Hom. name) cannot be traced and is probably trivial.

Sumbul see *Ferula sumbul*

Swertia chirata Buch.-Ham. ex Wall., Numer. List n. 4372. 1831.
Gentianaceae SWER-CH. Hn R
Chirata is the vernacular name and Chirata indica (Hom. name) is untraced.

Symphoricarpos albus (L.) Blake, Rhodora 16(187): 118. 1914.
Caprifoliaceae SYM-R. R
Vaccinium album L., Sp. Pl. 1: 350. 1753.
Symphoricarpos racemosus Michx., Fl. Bor.-Amer. ed. 1, 1: 107. 1803. Hn A

Symphoricarpos racemosus see *Symphoricarpos albus*

Symphytum officinale L., Sp. Pl. 1: 136. 1753.
Boraginaceae SYMPH. Hn R A F

Symplocarpus foetidus (L.) W. Salisb., Trans. Hort. Soc. London 1: 267. 1812, not (L.) Nutt.1818.
Araceae ICTOD. R A
Dracontium foetidum L., Sp. Pl. 2: 967. 1753.
Pothos foetidus (L.) Michx., Fl. Bor.-Amer. ed. 1, 2: 186. 1803, nom. illeg., "foetida", not Aiton 1789. Hs A
Ictodes foetidus Bigelow, Amer. Med. Bot. 2(1): 41. t. 24. 1819, incertae sedis.
Ictodes "foetida" (Hom. name) is an orthographic variant.

Syzygium cumini (L.) Skeels, U. S. D. A. Bur. Pl. Industr. Bull. 248: 25. 1912.
Myrtaceae SYZYG. Hs
Myrtus cumini L., Sp. Pl. 1: 471. 1753.
Syzygium jambolanum (Lam.) DC., Prodr. 3: 259. Mar 1828. Hn A
Eugenia jambolana Lam., Encycl. 3(1): 198. 1789. R
Eugenia "jambolanum" (Amer. Pharm.) is an orthographic variant.

Syzygium jambolanum see *Syzygium cumini*

Syzygium jambos (L.) Alston, Handb. Fl. Ceylon 6: 115. 1931.
Myrtaceae EUG. R
Eugenia jambos L., Sp. Pl. 1: 470. 1753. Hn A
Myrtus jambos (L.) Kunth, Nov. Gen. Sp. 6: 144. 1823. A
Jambos vulgaris DC., Prodr. 3: 286. Mar 1828.
"Jambosa" vulgaris (Hom. syn.) is a typographic error.

Tabacum see *Nicotiana tabacum*

Tamarindus indica L., Sp. Pl. 1: 34. 1753.
Fabaceae TAMA. Hn R

Tamus communis L., Sp. Pl. 2: 1028. 1753.
Dioscoreaceae TAM. Hn R A

Tanacetum parthenium (L.) Sch. Bip., Tanaceteen 55. 1844.
Asteraceae PYRE-P. R
Matricaria parthenium L., Sp. Pl. 2: 890. 1753.
Pyrethrum parthenium (L.) Sm., Fl. Brit. 2: 900. 1800. Hn

Tanacetum vulgare L., Sp. Pl. 2: 844. 1753.
Asteraceae TANAC. Hn R A
Chrysanthemum vulgare (L.) Bernh. Gaterau Syst. Verz. 144. 1800, nom. illeg. not Lam. 1789. G

Tanghinia venenifera see *Cerbera manghas*

Taraktogenos kurzii see *Hydnocarpus kurzii*

Taraxacum dens-leonis see *Taraxacum officinale*

Taraxacum officinale Weber, Prim. Fl. Holsat. 56. 1780.
Asteraceae TARAX. Hn R G A
Taraxacum dens-leonis Desf., Fl. Atlant. 2: 228. 1799.
Leontodon taraxacum L., Sp. Pl. 2: 798. 1753. Hs A
Dens leonis sensu Amer. Pharm., is pre-Linnaean.

Taxodium sempervirens see *Sequoia sempervirens*

Taxus baccata var. brevifolia see *Taxus brevifolia*

Taxus baccata L., Sp. Pl. 2: 1040. 1753.
Taxaceae TAX. Hn R G A

Taxus brevifolia Nutt., N. Amer. Sylv. 3: 86, t. 108. 1852.
Taxaceae TAX-BR. Hn R
Taxus baccata subsp. *brevifolia* (Nutt.) Pilg., Pflanzenr. IV. 5 (Heft 18): 113. 1903.
Taxus baccata L. var. *brevifolia* (Nutt.) Koehne, Deut. Dendrol. 6. 1893.

Terminalia arjuna (Roxb.) Wight & Arn., Prodr. Fl. Ind. Orient. 314. 1834.
Combretaceae TERM-A. Hn R
Pentaptera arjuna Roxb., Fl. Ind. 2: 438. 1832.

Terminalia chebula Retz., Observ. Bot. 5: 31. 1789.
Combretaceae TERM-C. Hn R

Tetranthera californica see *Umbellularia californica*

Teucrium marum L., Sp. Pl. 2: 564. 1753.
Lamiaceae TEUCR. Hn R G A
Linnaeus (1749 p. 100) uses Marum verum (Amer. Pharm.) as the medicinal name for *Teucrium marum*.

Teucrium scorodonia L., Sp. Pl. 2: 564. 1753.
Lamiaceae TEUCR-S. Hn R G F

Thapsus barbatus see *Verbascum thapsus*

Thea sinensis see *Camellia sinensis*

Theobroma augusta see *Ambroma augusta*

Theobroma cacao L., Sp. Pl. 2: 782. 1753.
Sterculiaceae CAC. R
Linnaeus (1749 p. 128) uses Cacao (Hom. name) as the medicinal name for *Theobroma cacao*.

Thevetia neriifolia see *Thevetia peruviana*

Thevetia peruviana (Pers.) K. Schum., Nat. Pflanzenfam. 4(2): 159. 1895.
Apocynaceae THEV.
Cerbera peruviana Pers., Syn. Pl. 1: 267. 1805.
Thevetia neriifolia Juss. ex Steud., Nomencl. Bot. ed. 2(2): 680. 1841. Hn R
Cerbera thevetia L., Sp. Pl. 1: 209. 1753. Hs

Thlaspi bursa-pastoris see *Capsella bursa-pastoris*

Thryallis glauca (Cav.) Kuntze, Revis. Gen. Pl. 1: 89. 1891.
Malpighiaceae GALPH. G
Galphimia glauca Cav., Icon. 5: 61, t. 489. 1799. Hn R
Galphimia gracilis Bartl., Linnaea 13: 552. 1840. Hs

Thuja lobbii see *Thuja plicata*

Thuja lobii see *Thuja plicata*

Thuja occidentalis L., Sp. Pl. 2: 1002. 1753.
Cupressaceae THUJ. Hn R G A F

Thuja plicata Donn ex D. Don, Descr. Pinus 2: 19. 1824.
Cupressaceae THUJ-L. Hs
Thuja lobbii Hort. ex Gordon, Pinetum 323. 1858, incertae sedis.
Thuja "lobii" (Comp. Rep.) is a typographic error.

Thymus serpyllum L., Sp. Pl. 2: 590. 1753.
Lamiaceae THYMU. Hn R G A

Tiangius pepetia see *Alternanthera repens*

Tiglium officinale see *Croton tiglium*

Tilia cordata Mill., Gard. Dict. ed. 8. "Tilia" 1. 1768.
Tiliaceae TIL-C. R

Tinospora cordifolia (Willd.) Miers, Ann. Mag. Nat. Hist. ser. 2, 7: 35, 38. 1851.
   Menispermaceae TINOS. Hn R
   Menispermum cordifolium Willd., Willd., Sp. Pl. 4(2): 826. 1805.

Toluifera balsamum see *Myroxylon balsamum*

Tongo see *Dipteryx odorata*

Tormentilla erecta see *Potentilla erecta*

Torula cerevisiae see *Saccharomyces cerevisiae*

Toxicodendron altissima see *Ailanthus altissima*

Toxicodendron diversilobum (Torr. & A. Gray) Greene, Leafl. Bot. Observ. Crit. 1:119. 1905.
   Anacardiaceae RHUS-D.
   Rhus diversiloba Torr. & A. Gray, Fl. N. Amer. 1(2): 218. 1838. Hn R
   Toxicodendron radicans subsp. *diversiloba* (Torr. & A. Gray) Thorne, Aliso 6(3): 28. 1967. R

Toxicodendron pubescens Mill., Gard. Dict. ed. 8. "Toxicodendron" 2. 1768.
   Anacardiaceae RHUS-T.
   Rhus verrucosa Scheele, Linnaea 21: 592. 1848. A
   Rhus toxicodendron L., Sp. Pl. 1: 266. 1753. R A F
   Incorrect usage: *Rhus radicans* (Hom. name and Amer. Pharm.), not L.

Toxicodendron radicans subsp. diversiloba see *Toxicodendron diversilobum*

Toxicodendron radicans (L.) Kuntze, Revis. Gen. Pl. 1: 153. 1891.
   Anacardiaceae RHUS-R. R
   Rhus radicans L., Sp. Pl. 1: 266. 1753. Hn

Toxicodendron vernix (L.) Kuntze, Revis. Gen. Pl. 1: 153. 1891.
   Anacardiaceae RHUS-V. R
   Rhus vernix L., Sp. Pl. 1: 265. 1753. A
   Rhus venenata DC., Prodr. 2: 68. Nov 1825. Hn A

Toxicophlaea thunbergii Harv., London J. Bot. 1: 24. 1842.
   Apocynaceae TOX-TH.
   "Toxicophloea thunbergi" (Comp. Rep.) is a typographic error.

Toxicophloea thunbergi see *Toxicophlaea thunbergii*

Tradescantia diuretica see *Tripogandra diuretica*

Tribulus terrestris L., Sp. Pl. 1: 387. 1753.
   Zygophyllaceae TRIB. Hn R

Trichosanthes dioica Roxb., Fl. Ind. ed. 1832. 3: 701. 1832.
   Cucurbitaceae TRICH-D. Hn R

Trifolium campestre see *Trifolium pratense*

Trifolium melilotus var. officinalis see *Melilotus officinalis*

Trifolium officinale see *Melilotus officinalis*

Trifolium pratense L., Sp. Pl. 2: 768. 1753.
Fabaceae TRIF-P. Hn R A
Incorrect usage: *Trifolium campestre* sensu Amer. pharm., not Schreb., and *Trifolium procumbens* sensu Amer. Pharm., not L.

Trifolium procumbens see *Trifolium pratense*

Trifolium repens L., Sp. Pl. 2: 767. 1753.
Fabaceae TRIF-R. Hn R A

Trillium cernuum L, Sp. Pl. 1: 339. 1753, not W. P. C. Barton 1821.
Trilliaceae TRIL-C. Hn R A
Incorrect usage: *Trillium pendulum* sensu Amer. Pharm., not Willd.

Trillium erectum L., Sp. Pl. 1: 340. 1753.
Trilliaceae TRIL. Hn R
Trillium pendulum Willd., Ges. Naturf. Freunde Berlin Neue Schriften 3: 421. 1801, incertae sedis. Hs

Trillium pendulum see *Trillium erectum* and *Trillium cernuum*

Trimezia galaxioides (Gomes) Ravenna, Wrightia 7(2): 94. 1982.
Iridaceae SISY.
Sisyrinchium galaxioides Gomes, Mem. Math. Phis. Acad. Real Sci. Lisboa 3. 1812; Mem. Corresp. 99. {The date of publication could be 1814} Hn R
Sisyrinchium "galaxoides" (Comp. Rep.) is a typographic error.

Triosteum perfoliatum L., Sp. Pl. 1: 176. 1753.
Caprifoliaceae TRIO. Hn R A

Tripogandra diuretica (Mart.) Handlos, Rhodora 77(810): 259. 1975.
Commelinaceae TRAD. Hn R
Tradescantia diuretica Mart., Reise Bras. 281. 1823.

Triticum repens see *Agropyron repens*

Tropaeolum majus L., Sp. Pl. 1: 345. 1753.
Tropaeolaceae TROP. Hn R F

Tsuga canadensis (L.) Carrière, Traité Gén. Conif. 189. 1855.
Pinaceae ABIES-C. Hs
Pinus canadensis L., Sp. Pl. ed. 2. 1421. 1763. A
Abies canadensis (L.) Michx., Fl. Bor.-Amer. ed. 1, 2: 206. 1803. nom. illeg, not Mill. 1768. Hn R G A

Tulipa breyniana see *Homeria breyniana*

Turnera aphrodisiaca see *Turnera diffusa*

Turnera diffusa Willd. ex Schult., Syst. Veg. 6: 679. 1820.
Turneraceae DAM. Hs G F
Turnera diffusa var. *aphrodisiaca* (Ward) Urb., Jahrb. Königl. Bot. Gart. Berlin 2: 127. 1883. Hs G F

Turnera aphrodisiaca Ward, Virg. Med. Monthly 49. 1876. ex J. Bot. 18: 20. 1880. R F
Common homeopathic name: Damiana. The German pharmacopoeia uses *Turnera diffusa* and its varieties for the preparation of the remedy.

Turnera diffusa var. aphrodisiaca see *Turnera diffusa*

Tussilago farfara L., Sp. Pl. 2: 865. 1753.
Asteraceae TUS-FA. Hn R

Tussilago fragrans see *Petasites fragrans*

Tussilago hybrida see *Petasites hybridus*

Tussilago petasites see *Petasites hybridus*

Tylophora indica (Burm. f.) Merr., Philipp. J. Sci. 19: 373. 1921.
Asclepiadaceae TYLO-I. Hn R
Cynanchum indicum Burm. f., Fl. Indica 70. 1768.

Typha latifolia L., Sp. Pl. 2: 971. 1753.
Typhaceae TYPH. Hn R

Ulmus fulva see *Ulmus rubra*

Ulmus rubra Muhl., Trans. Amer. Philos. Soc. 5: 169. 1793.
Ulmaceae ULM.
Ulmus fulva Michx., Fl. Bor.-Amer. ed. 1, 1: 172. 1803. Hn R

Umbellularia californica (Hook. & Arn.) Nutt., N. Amer. Sylv. 1: 87. 1852.
Lauraceae OREO. R
Tetranthera californica Hook. & Arn., Bot. Beechey Voy 159. 1833.
Oreodaphne californica (Hook. & Arn.) Nees, Syst. Laur. 465. 1836. Hn

Umbilicus pendulinus see *Cotyledon umbilicus*

Upas antiaris see *Antiaris toxicaria*

Upas tieute see *Strychnos tieute*

Uredo maydis see *Ustilago maydis*

Urginea maritima see *Drimia maritima*

Urtica crenulata see *Dendrocnide sinuata*

Urtica gigas see *Laportea gigas*

Urtica sinuata see *Dendrocnide sinuata*

Urtica urens L., Sp. Pl. 2: 984. 1753.
Urticaceae URT-U. Hn R A F

Usnea barbata (L.) Weber ex F. H. Wigg., Prim. Fl. Holsat. 91. 1780.
Parmeliaceae USN. Hn R A
Lichen barbatus L., Sp. Pl. 2: 1155. 1753.

Ustilago maydis (DC.) Corda., Icon. Fung. 5: 3. 1842.

Ustilaginaceae UST. R A F
Uredo maydis DC., Fl. Franç. 6: 77. 1815.
Ustilago zeae Unger, Einfl. Boden. Verth. Gew. 211. 1836. G
Corn-smut (Hom. name) is the common name for *Ustilago maydis*.

Ustilago zeae see *Ustilago maydis*

Uva-ursi see *Arctostaphylos uva-ursi*

Uvaria triloba see *Asimina triloba*

Vaccinium album see *Symphoricarpos albus*

Vaccinium myrtillus L., Sp. Pl. 1: 349. 1753.
Ericaceae VACC-M. Hn R G F

Valeriana officinalis L., Sp. Pl. 1: 31. 1753.
Valerianaceae VALER. Hn R G A F

Vanilla planifolia Jacks. ex Andrews, Bot. Repos. 8: t. 538. 1808.
Orchidaceae VANIL. Hn R

Vataireopsis araroba (Aguiar) Ducke, Ann. Acad. Brasil. Sci. 8: 26. 1936.
Fabaceae CHRYSAR.
Andira araroba Aguiar, Gazeta Medica da Bahia 10(8): 353. 1878. {Publication not seen} R
Chrysarobinum is the homeopathic name for Chrysarobin, the substance obtained by extraction from the trunk of *Andira araroba*.

Veratrum album L., Sp. Pl. 2: 1044. 1753.
Melanthiaceae VERAT. Hn R A F

Veratrum luteum see *Helonias dioica*

Veratrum nigrum L., Sp. Pl. 2: 1044. 1753.
Melanthiaceae VERAT-N. Hn R A

Veratrum officinale see *Schoenocaulon officinale*

Veratrum viride see *Helonias viridis*

Verbascum thapsiforme see *Verbascum thapsus*

Verbascum thapsus L., Sp. Pl. 1: 177. 1753.
Scrophulariaceae VERB. Hn R A F
Verbascum thapsiforme Guss., Fl. Sicul. Prodr. 1: 262. 1827, not Schrad. 1813. G
Thapsus barbatus Bedevian, lllustr. Polyglot. Dict. 609. 1936. A
Incorrect usage: *Verbascum thapsiforme* sensu Germ. Pharm., not Schrad.

Verbena hastata L., Sp. Pl. 1: 20. 1753.
Verbenaceae VERBE-H. Hn R A

Verbena urticifolia L., Sp. Pl. 1: 20. 1753.
Verbcnaceae VERBE-U. Hn R

Verbena verticillata see *Vitex agnus-castus*

Vernonia anthelmintica (L.) Willd., Willd., Sp. Pl. 3(3): 1634. 1803.
Asteraceae VERN-A. Hn R
Conyza anthelmintica L., Sp. Pl. ed. 2. 1207. 1763.

Veronica americana see *Veronica beccabunga*

Veronica beccabunga L., Sp. Pl. 1: 12. 1753.
Scrophulariaceae VERO-B. Hn R A
Incorrect usage: *Veronica americana* sensu Amer. Pharm., not Schwein. ex Benth.

Veronica virginica see *Veronicastrum virginicum*

Veronicastrum virginicum (L.) Farw., Druggists Circular, 61: 231. 1917, as cited by Pennell in Rhodora, 23: 6. 1921
Scrophulariaceae LEPT.
Veronica virginica L., Sp. Pl. 1: 9. 1753. R Hs G A
Leptandra virginica (L.) Nutt., Gen. N. Amer. Pl. 1: 7. 1818. Hn

Vetivera zizanoides see *Vetiveria zizanioides*

Vetiveria zizanioides (L.) Nash, Fl. S.E. U.S. 67, 1326. 1903.
Poaceae ANAN.
Phalaris zizanioides L., Mant. Pl. 2: 183. 1771.
Andropogon squarrosus L. f., Suppl. Pl. 433. 1782. Hs
Andropogon muricatus Retz., Observ. Bot. 3: 43. 1783. R A
Andropogon muricatum Retz., Observ. Bot. 3: 43. 1783.
Anatherum muricatum (Retz.) P. Beauv., Ess. Agrostogr. 150, Atlas 15, t. 22, f. 10. 1812, nom. nud.
"Anantherum" muricatum (Hom. name) and *"Vetivera zizanoides"* (Hom. syn.) is a typograhic error.

Viborquia polystachya see *Eysenhardtia polystachya*

Viburnum odoratissimum Ker Gawl., Bot. Reg. 6: t. 456. 1820.
Caprifoliaceae VIB-OD. Hn R

Viburnum opulus L., Sp. Pl. 1: 268. 1753.
Caprifoliaceae VIB. Hn R G A

Viburnum prunifolium L., Sp. Pl. 1: 268. 1753.
Caprifoliaceae VIB-P. Hn R A F

Viburnum tinus L., Sp. Pl. 1: 267. 1753.
Caprifoliaceae VIB-T. Hn R

Vinca minor L., Sp. Pl. 1: 209. 1753.
Apocynaceae VINC. Hn R G A F

Vincetoxicum hirundinaria Medik., Hist. & Commentat. Acad. Elect. Sci. Theod.-Palat. 6: 404. 1790.
Asclepiadaceae VINCE. G
Vincetoxicum officinale Moench, Methodus 717. 1794, nom. illeg. Hn R

Vincetoxicum officinale see *Vincetoxicum hirundinaria*

Viola alba see *Viola odorata*

Viola odorata L., Sp. Pl. 2: 934. 1753.
 Violaceae VIOL-O. Hn R A
 Incorrect usage: *Viola alba* sensu Amer. Pharm., not Besser.

Viola tricolor L., Sp. Pl. 2: 935. 1753.
 Violaceae VIOL-T. Hn R G A F

Virola sebifera see *Myristica sebifera*

Viscum album L., Sp. Pl. 2: 1023. 1753.
 Viscaceae VISC. Hn R G A F

Vitex agnus-castus L., Sp. Pl. 2: 638. 1753.
 Verbenaceae AGN. R G A F
 Linnaeus (1749 p. 112) uses Agnus castus (Hom. name) as the medicinal name. *Verbena verticillata* (Hom. syn.) is an untraced name.

Vitex trifolia L., Sp. Pl. 2: 638. 1753.
 Verbenaceae VIT. Hn R

Warneria canadensis see *Hydrastis canadensis*

Wigandia californica see *Eriodictyon californicum*

Wyethia helenioides (DC.) Nutt., Trans. Amer. Philos. Soc., n.s., 7: 353. 1840.
 Asteraceae WYE. Hn R A
 Alarconia helenioides DC., Prodr. 5: 537. Oct 1836.

Xanthium spinosum L., Sp. Pl. 2: 987. 1753.
 Asteraceae XANTH. Hn R

Xanthorhiza apiifolia L'Hér., Stirp. Nov. fasc. 4. 79. 1788.
 Ranunculaceae XANRHI. Hn R

Xanthorrhoea arborea R. Br., Prodr. ed. 1, 288. 1810.
 Xanthorrhoeacea XANRHOE. Hn R

Xanthoxylum americanum see *Zanthoxylum americanum*

Yucca filamentosa L., Sp. Pl. 1: 319. 1753.
 Agavaceae YUC. Hn R A F

Zamia spiralis see *Macrozamia spiralis*

Zanthoxylum americanum Mill., Gard. Dict. ed. 8. "Zanthoxylum" 2. 1768.
 Rutaceae XAN. R
 "Xanthoxylum" americanum (Hom. name) is an orthographic variant.

Zapania scaberrima see *Phyla scaberrima*

Zea italica see *Zea mays*

Zea mays L., Sp. Pl. 2: 971. 1753.
 Poaceae ZEA-I.

Zea italica (Comp. Rep., and Hom. name) is an unknown combination. A separate remedy Stigmata maydis (Comp. Rep., and Hom. name).abbreviated to STIGM, is made from the "green pistils" of *Zea mays*.

Zingiber officinale Roscoe, Trans. Linn. Soc. London 8: 348. 1807.
Zingiberaceae ZING. Hn R G A F

Zizia aurea (L.) Koch, Nova Acta Phys.-Med. Acad. Caes. Leop.-Carol. Nat. Cur. 12(I): 129. 1824.
Apiaceae ZIZ. Hn R
Smyrnium aureum L., Sp. Pl. 1: 262. 1753.

Zygophyllum tridentatum see *Larrea tridentata*

Untraced names

The names below are either untraceable or of unknown combinations. Where possible an explanation of their status or closest name match is given.

Aegle folia Rutaceae AEGLE-F
  This remedy is made from the leaves of *Aegle marmelos,* which already exists as a separate remedy. See AEGLE.

Dialium ferrum Fabaceae DIAL.
  Dialium is a valid generic name but the combination Dialium ferrum is unknown.

Dichapetalum thunbergh Dichapetalaceae DICHA.
  Dichapetalum is a valid generic name but the combination is untraceable.

Illecebrum Caryophyllaceae ILLEC.
  This could be the generic name and one of several species or could be the specific epithet, which by itself has no standing. In either case the name is ambiguous.

Iris factissima Iridaceae IRIS-FA.
  The closest name match is *Iris flavissima* Pall.

Melastoma ackermani Melastomaceae MELA.

Myosotis symphytifolia Boraginaceae MYOS.

Panacea arvensis Dryopteridaceae PANA.

Pinus cupressus Pinaceae PIN-C.

Plumeria celinus Apocynaceae PLUME.

Quercus glandibus Fagaceae QUERC.
  The closest possible name match is *Quercus glandulifera* Blume.

Silphion cyrenaicum Asteraceae SILPHO.

Vesicaria communis Brassicaceae VESI.

Viscum quercinum Viscaceae **visc-q**.

Vitrum antimonii Poaceae **vitr**.
> Likely to be a mistake for glass = vitrum or maybe an obscure reference to *Salicornia* spp.(glasswort).

Xerophyllum Melanthiaceae **xero**.
> As in the case of Illecebrum this name is ambiguous as it does not specify which species was used in the preparation of the remedy.

Index by Family Names

This list provides all family names arranged alphabetically with their accepted species. The names of vascular plants follow the system adopted by Brummitt, *Vascular Plant Families and Genera*, 1992 and for most Fungi and Lichens the *Dictionary of Fungi*, 1995 by Ainsworth and Bisby. All family names conform to standard usage and end with *-aceae*. The only exceptions are eight families that have two alternative names. The alternative names are cited in parenthesis: Apiaceae (Umbelliferae); Arecaceae (Palmae); Asteraceae (Compositae); Brassicaceae (Cruciferae); Clusiaceae (Guttiferae); Fabaceae (Leguminosae); Lamiaceae (Labiatae) and Poaceae (Gramineae).

Acanthaceae
Adhatoda vasica
Andrographis paniculata
Odontonema rubrum

Aceraceae
Acer negundo

Adoxaceae
Adoxa moschatellina

Agaricaceae (Eumycota [Fungi])
Agaricus campestris
Macrolepiota procera

Agavaceae
Agave americana
Agave tequilana
Yucca filamentosa

Alliaceae
Allium cepa
Allium sativum

Aloeaceae
Aloe succotrina

Amanitaceae (Eumycota [Fungi])
Amanita citrina
Amanita muscaria
Amanita pantherina
Amanita phalloides

Amaranthaceae
Achyranthes aspera
Alternanthera repens
Iresine calea

Amaryllidaceae
Galanthus nivalis

Narcissus poeticus
Narcissus pseudonarcissus

Anacardiaceae
Amphipterygium adstringens
Anacardium occidentale
Comocladia dentata
Malosma laurina
Mangifera indica
Rhus aromatica
Rhus glabra
Schinus molle
Semecarpus anacardium
Toxicodendron diversilobum
Toxicodendron pubescens
Toxicodendron radicans
Toxicodendron vernix

Annonaceae
Asimina triloba
Guatteria gaumeri

Apiaceae (Umbelliferae)
Aegopodium podagraria
Aethusa cynapium
Angelica atropurpurea
Angelica sinensis
Apium graveolens
Centella asiatica
Cicuta maculata
Cicuta virosa
Conium maculatum
Dorema ammoniacum
Eryngium aquaticum
Eryngium maritimum
Ferula communis
Ferula narthex
Ferula sumbul
Heracleum sphondylium
Oenanthe aquatica
Oenanthe crocata
Pastinaca sativa
Petroselinum crispum
Peucedanum oreoselinum
Peucedanum ostruthium
Pimpinella saxifraga
Sium latifolium
Zizia aurea

Apocynaceae
Acokanthera schimperi

Alstonia constricta
Alstonia scholaris
Apocynum androsaemifolium
Apocynum cannabinum
Cerbera manghas
Echites suberecta
Holarrhena pubescens
Macaglia quebracho-blanco
Nerium oleander
Rauwolfia serpentina
Strophanthus kombe
Strophanthus sarmentosus
Thevetia peruviana
Toxicophlaea thunbergii
Vinca minor

Aquifoliaceae
Ilex aquifolium
Ilex cassine
Ilex paraguariensis

Araceae
Amorphophallus konjac
Arisaema dracontium
Arisaema triphyllum
Arum italicum
Arum maculatum
Dieffenbachia seguine
Dracunculus vulgaris
Symplocarpus foetidus

Araliaceae
Aralia hispida
Aralia quinquefolia
Aralia racemosa
Hedera helix

Arecaceae (Palmae)
Areca catechu
Elaeis guineensis
Lodoicea maldivica
Serenoa repens

Aristolochiaceae
Aristolochia clematitis
Aristolochia cymbifera
Aristolochia serpentaria
Asarum canadense
Asarum europaeum

Asclepiadaceae
Asclepias incarnata

Asclepias syriaca
Asclepias tuberosa
Calotropis gigantea
Gymnema sylvestre
Marsdenia cundurango
Periploca graeca
Tylophora indica
Vincetoxicum hirundinaria

Asparagaceae
Asparagus officinalis

Aspleniaceae
Asplenium scolopendrium

Asteraceae (Compositae)
Achillea millefolium
Ageratina aromatica
Ambrosia artemisiifolia
Arctium lappa
Arnica montana
Artemisia abrotanum
Artemisia absinthium
Artemisia vulgaris
Bellis perennis
Blumea balsamifera
Brachyglottis repanda
Calea ternifolia
Calendula officinalis
Centaurea tagana
Chamaemelum nobile
Cichorium intybus
Cnicus benedictus
Conyza canadensis
Cynara cardunculus
Echinacea angustifolia
Echinacea purpurea
Erechtites hieracifolia
Espeletia grandiflora
Eupatorium perfoliatum
Eupatorium purpureum
Galinsoga parviflora
Gnaphalium polycephalum
Grindelia rubricaulis var. *robusta*
Haplopappus baylahuen
Helianthus annuus
Hieracium pilosella
Inula helenium
Lactuca virosa
Lapsana communis

Leucanthemum vulgare
Liatris spicata
Matricaria recutita
Mikania amara var. *guaco*
Nabalus serpentarius
Onopordum acanthium
Parthenium hysterophorus
Petasites fragrans
Petasites hybridus
Polymnia uvedalia
Senecio aureus
Senecio bicolor subsp. *cineraria*
Senecio jacobaea
Seriphidium maritimum
Sigesbeckia orientalis
Silphium laciniatum
Silybum marianum
Solidago virgaurea
Tanacetum parthenium
Tanacetum vulgare
Taraxacum officinale
Tussilago farfara
Vernonia anthelmintica
Wyethia helenioides
Xanthium spinosum

Balanophoraceae
Lophophytum leandrii

Berberidaceae
Berberis vulgaris
Caulophyllum thalictroides
Mahonia aquifolium
Podophyllum peltatum

Betulaceae
Alnus serrulata
Ostrya virginiana

Bignoniaceae
Catalpa bignonioides
Jacaranda caroba
Jacaranda mimosifolia

Bixaceae
Bixa orellana

Boletaceae (Eumycota [Fungi])
Boletus luridus
Boletus satanas

Boraginaceae

Borago officinalis
Heliotropium arborescens
Myosotis arvensis
Onosmodium virginianum
Symphytum officinale

Brassicaceae (Cruciferae)
Armoracia rusticana
Brassica alba
Brassica napus
Brassica nigra
Brassica oleracea
Bunias orientalis
Capsella bursa-pastoris
Cheiranthus cheiri
Cochlearia officinalis
Iberis amara
Lepidium bonariense
Matthiola incana
Raphanus sativus
Rorippa nasturtium-aquaticum

Buxaceae
Buxus sempervirens

Cactaceae
Cereus serpentinus
Harrisia bonplandii
Lophophora williamsii var. *lewinii*
Opuntia ficus-indica
Opuntia microdasys
Opuntia vulgaris
Selenicereus grandiflorus

Campanulaceae
Lobelia cardinalis
Lobelia colorata
Lobelia dortmanna
Lobelia erinus
Lobelia inflata
Lobelia siphilitica

Cannabaceae
Cannabis indica
Cannabis sativa
Humulus lupulus

Cannaceae
Canna glauca

Capparaceae
Capparis coriacea

Caprifoliaceae
Lonicera caprifolium
Lonicera periclymenum
Lonicera xylosteum
Sambucus canadensis
Sambucus nigra
Symphoricarpos albus
Triosteum perfoliatum
Viburnum odoratissimum
Viburnum opulus
Viburnum prunifolium
Viburnum tinus

Caricaceae
Carica papaya

Caryophyllaceae
Agrostemma githago
Saponaria officinalis
Stellaria media

Cecropiaceae
Cecropia obtusifolia

Celastraceae
Euonymus atropurpureus
Euonymus europaea

Chenopodiaceae
Atriplex hortensis
Beta vulgaris
Chenopodium ambrosioides
Chenopodium vulvaria

Cistaceae
Helianthemum canadense

Clavicipitaceae (Eumycota [Fungi])
Claviceps purpurea

Clusiaceae (Guttiferae)
Garcinia morella
Hypericum perforatum

Colchicaceae
Colchicum autumnale

Combretaceae
Terminalia arjuna
Terminalia chebula

Commelinaceae
Tripogandra diuretica

Compositae see *Asteraceae*

Convallariaceae
Convallaria majalis

Convolvulaceae
Calystegia spithamaea subsp. *stans*
Convolvulus arvensis
Convolvulus scammonia
Ipomoea alba
Ipomoea purga
Ipomoea purpurea
Operculina turpethum

Coprinaceae (Eumycota [Fungi])
Coprinus stercorarius

Coriariaceae
Coriaria myrtifolia
Coriaria ruscifolia

Coriolaceae (Eumycota [Fungi])
Fomitopsis officinalis
Fomitopsis pinicola

Cornaceae
Cornus alternifolia
Cornus circinata
Cornus florida
Cornus sericea

Corynocarpaceae
Corynocarpus laevigatus

Crassulaceae
Cotyledon umbilicus
Hylotelephium telephium
Sedum acre
Sedum alpestre
Sempervivum tectorum

Cruciferae see *Brassicaceae*

Cucurbitaceae
Bryonia alba
Citrullus colocynthis
Citrullus lanatus
Coccinia grandis
Cucurbita pepo
Ecballium elaterium
Luffa amara
Luffa bondel
Luffa operculata

Momordica balsamina
Momordica charantia
Trichosanthes dioica

Cupressaceae
Chamaecyparis lawsoniana
Juniperus communis
Juniperus sabina
Juniperus virginiana
Thuja occidentalis
Thuja plicata

Dioscoreaceae
Dioscorea villosa
Tamus communis

Droseraceae
Drosera rotundifolia

Dryopteridaceae
Dryopteris filix-mas

Ephedraceae
Ephedra distachya

Equisetaceae
Equisetum arvense
Equisetum hyemale

Ericaceae
Arbutus andrachne
Arbutus menziesii
Arctostaphylos pungens
Arctostaphylos uva-ursi
Chimaphila maculata
Chimaphila umbellata
Epigaea repens
Gaultheria procumbens
Kalmia latifolia
Ledum palustre
Oxydendrum arboreum
Rhododendron aureum
Vaccinium myrtillus

Erythroxylaceae
Erythroxylum coca

Euphorbiaceae
Acalypha indica
Chamaesyce prostrata
Cnidoscolus urens
Croton eluteria
Croton tiglium

Euphorbia amygdaloides
Euphorbia corollata
Euphorbia cyparissias
Euphorbia heterodoxa
Euphorbia hirta
Euphorbia hypericifolia
Euphorbia ipecacuanhae
Euphorbia lathyrus
Euphorbia officinarum
Euphorbia peplus
Euphorbia polycarpa
Hippomane mancinella
Hura crepitans
Jatropha curcas
Mallotus philippensis
Manihot esculenta
Mercurialis perennis
Ricinus communis
Stillingia sylvatica

Fabaceae (Leguminosae)
Abrus precatorius
Anagyris foetida
Astragalus exscapus
Astragalus nuttallii
Baptisia australis
Baptisia tinctoria
Caesalpinia bonduc
Calliandra houstoniana
Cassia fistula
Copaifera officinalis
Cytisus scoparius
Dalbergia pinnata
Desmodium barbatum
Desmodium gangeticum
Dipteryx odorata
Erythrophleum suaveolens
Eysenhardtia polystachya
Galega officinalis
Genista tinctoria
Gymnocladus dioica
Haematoxylum campechianum
Indigofera tinctoria
Laburnum anagyroides
Lathyrus sativus
Medicago sativa
Melilotus albus
Melilotus officinalis
Mimosa dormiens

Mimosa pudica
Mimosa quadrivalvis var. *angusta*
Mucuna pruriens
Mucuna urens
Myroxylon balsamum
Myroxylon balsamum var. *pereirae*
Ononis spinosa
Oxytropis lambertii
Phaseolus vulgaris
Physostigma venenosum
Piscidia piscipula
Psoralea bituminosa
Robinia pseudoacacia
Saraca asoca
Senna alexandrina
Senna sophera
Tamarindus indica
Trifolium pratense
Trifolium repens
Vataireopsis araroba

Fagaceae
Castanea sativa
Fagus sylvatica
Quercus robur

Flacourtiaceae
Hydnocarpus kurzii

Fucophyceae (Phaeophyta [Brown Algae])
Fucus vesiculosus

Fumariaceae
Fumaria officinalis

Gentianaceae
Centaurium chironioides
Gentiana cruciata
Gentiana lutea
Gentianella quinquefolia
Swertia chirata

Geraniaceae
Erodium cicutarium
Geranium maculatum
Monsonia emarginata
Pelargonium reniforme

Ginkgoaceae
Ginkgo biloba

Gramineae see *Poaceae*

Guttiferae see *Clusiaceae*

Haemodoraceae
Lachnanthes caroliniana

Hamamelidaceae
Hamamelis virginiana

Hippocastanaceae
Aesculus glabra
Aesculus hippocastanum

Hyacinthaceae
Drimia maritima
Hyacinthoides non-scripta
Ornithogalum umbellatum

Hydrangeaceae
Hydrangea arborescens

Hydrophyllaceae
Eriodictyon californicum
Hydrophyllum virginianum

Illecebraceae
Scleranthus annuus

Illiciaceae
Illicium anisatum

Iridaceae
Crocus sativus
Homeria breyniana
Iris florentina
Iris foetidissima
Iris germanica
Iris tenax
Iris versicolor
Trimezia galaxioides

Juglandaceae
Carya tomentosa
Juglans cinerea
Juglans regia

Juncaceae
Juncus effusus

Krameriaceae
Krameria lappacea

Labiatae see *Lamiaceae*

Lamiaceae (Labiatae)
Clerodendranthus stamineus

Collinsonia canadensis
Glechoma hederacea
Hedeoma pulegioides
Lamium album
Leonurus cardiaca
Lycopus virginicus
Marrubium vulgare
Mentha pulegium
Mentha spicata
Mentha x piperita
Micromeria chamissonis
Nepeta cataria
Ocimum canum
Ocimum caryophyllatum
Ocimum tenuiflorum
Origanum majorana
Origanum vulgare
Plectranthus amboinicus
Plectranthus fruticosus
Rosmarinus officinalis
Salvia officinalis
Salvia sclarea
Satureja hortensis
Scutellaria lateriflora
Stachys officinalis
Teucrium marum
Teucrium scorodonia
Thymus serpyllum

Lauraceae
Aniba coto
Cinnamomum camphora
Cinnamomum zeylanicum
Lindera benzoin
Nectandra amara
Persea americana
Umbellularia californica

Leguminosae see *Fabaceae*

Lemnaceae
Lemna minor

Liliaceae
Lilium lancifolium
Lilium superbum

Linaceae
Linum catharticum
Linum usitatissimum

Lobariaceae (Lichens)

Lobaria pulmonaria

Loganiaceae
Gelsemium sempervirens
Spigelia anthelmia
Spigelia marilandica
Strychnos axillaris
Strychnos ignatii
Strychnos nux-vomica
Strychnos tieute

Lycoperdaceae (Eumycota [Fungi])
Calvatia gigantea

Lycopodiaceae
Lycopodium clavatum

Lythraceae
Cuphea viscosissima
Punica granatum

Magnoliaceae
Magnolia grandiflora
Magnolia virginiana

Malpighiaceae
Banisteriopsis caapi
Thryallis glauca

Malvaceae
Abelmoschus moschatus
Althaea officinalis
Gossypium herbaceum

Melanthiaceae
Aletris farinosa
Helonias dioica
Helonias viridis
Schoenocaulon officinale
Veratrum album
Veratrum nigrum

Meliaceae
Azadirachta indica
Guarea guidonia

Menispermaceae
Anamirta cocculus
Chondrodendron tomentosum
Menispermum canadense
Tinospora cordifolia

Menyanthaceae
Menyanthes trifoliata

Metschnikowiaceae (Eumycota [Fungi])
Candida albicans

Monimiaceae
Peumus boldus

Moraceae
Antiaris toxicaria
Brosimum gaudichaudii
Ficus benghalensis
Ficus religiosa
Ficus tsjakela

Mucoraceae (Eumycota [Fungi])
Mucor mucedo

Musaceae
Musa sapientum

Myricaceae
Myrica cerifera

Myristicaceae
Myristica fragrans
Myristica sebifera

Myrsinaceae
Embelia ribes

Myrtaceae
Angophora costata subsp. *costata*
Eucalyptus globulus
Eucalyptus rostrata
Eucalyptus tereticornis
Luma chequen
Melaleuca cajuputi
Myrtus communis
Pimenta dioica
Syzygium cumini
Syzygium jambos

Nepenthaceae
Nepenthes distillatoria

Nyctaginaceae
Boerhavia diffusa

Nymphaeaceae
Nuphar lutea
Nymphaea odorata

Oleaceae
Chionanthus virginica
Fraxinus americana

Fraxinus excelsior
Jasminum officinale
Nyctanthes arbor-tristis

Onagraceae
Epilobium angustifolium
Epilobium palustre
Oenothera biennis

Orchidaceae
Corallorhiza odontorhiza
Cypripedium calceolus var. *pubescens*
Dipodium punctatum
Spiranthes spiralis
Vanilla planifolia

Oxalidaceae
Oxalis acetosella

Palmae see *Arecaceae*

Papaveraceae
Adlumia fungosa
Argemone mexicana
Chelidonium majus
Dicentra canadensis
Eschscholzia californica
Papaver somniferum
Sanguinaria canadensis

Parmeliaceae (Lichens)
Cetraria islandica
Usnea barbata

Passifloraceae
Passiflora incarnata

Pedaliceae
Harpagophytum procumbens

Penthoraceae
Penthorum sedoides

Phallaceae (Eumycota [Fungi])
Phallus impudicus

Phytolaccaceae
Petiveria alliacea var. *tetrandra*
Phytolacca americana

Pinaceae
Picea mariana
Pinus lambertiana
Pinus sylvestris

Pseudotsuga menziesii
Tsuga canadensis

Piperaceae
Piper aduncum
Piper cubeba
Piper methysticum
Piper nigrum

Plantaginaceae
Plantago major
Plantago minor

Platanaceae
Platanus x hispanica

Plumbaginaceae
Plumbago scandens

Poaceae (Gramineae)
Agropyron repens
Ampelodesmos mauritanica
Anthoxanthum odoratum
Avena sativa
Bambusa arundinacea
Cymbopogon citratus
Cynodon dactylon
Lolium temulentum
Phleum pratense
Saccharum officinarum
Vetiveria zizanioides
Zea mays

Polemoniaceae
Loeselia coccinea

Polygalaceae
Polygala senega

Polygonaceae
Fagopyrum esculentum
Polygonum aviculare
Polygonum persicaria
Polygonum punctatum
Polygonum sagittatum
Rheum palmatum
Rumex acetosa
Rumex crispus
Rumex obtusifolius

Polytrichaceae
Polytrichum juniperinum

Pontederiaceae
Eichhornia crassipes

Primulaceae
Anagallis arvensis
Androsace lactea
Cyclamen purpurascens
Lysimachia nummularia
Primula farinosa
Primula obconica
Primula veris

Ranunculaceae
Aconitum anthora
Aconitum ferox
Aconitum lycoctonum
Aconitum napellus
Aconitum septentrionale
Aconitum x cammarum
Actaea racemosa
Actaea spicata
Adonis vernalis
Aquilegia vulgaris
Caltha palustris
Clematis recta
Clematis vitalba
Delphinium staphisagria
Eranthis hyemalis
Helleborus foetidus
Helleborus niger
Helleborus orientalis
Helleborus viridis
Hepatica nobilis
Hydrastis canadensis
Paeonia officinalis
Pulsatilla patens
Pulsatilla pratensis
Ranunculus acris
Ranunculus bulbosus
Ranunculus flammula
Ranunculus glacialis
Ranunculus repens
Ranunculus sceleratus
Xanthorhiza apiifolia

Rhamnaceae
Ceanothus americanus
Ceanothus thyrsiflorus
Frangula alnus
Karwinskia humboldtiana

Rhamnus californica
Rhamnus cathartica
Rhamnus purshiana

Rhodomelaceae (Rhodophyta [Red Algae])
Alsidium helminthochorton

Rosaceae
Agrimonia eupatoria
Crataegus laevigata
Filipendula ulmaria
Fragaria vesca
Geum rivale
Hagenia abyssinica
Malus pumila
Potentilla anserina
Potentilla erecta
Prunus cerasifera
Prunus dulcis
Prunus laurocerasus
Prunus padus
Prunus persica
Prunus spinosa
Prunus virginiana
Pyrus americana
Quillaja saponaria
Rosa damascena
Sanguisorba officinalis

Rubiaceae
Cephalanthus occidentalis
Chiococca alba
Cinchona officinalis
Coffea arabica
Galium aparine
Galium odoratum
Mitchella repens
Psychotria ipecacuanha
Rubia tinctorum

Russulaceae (Eumycota [Fungi])
Russula emetica
Russula foetens

Rutaceae
Adenandra uniflora
Aegle marmelos
Agathosma crenulata
Angostura trifoliata
Brucea antidysenterica
Citrus maxima

Citrus x aurantium
Citrus x limon
Dictamnus albus
Glycosmis pentaphylla
Pilocarpus microphyllus
Ptelea trifoliata
Ruta graveolens
Zanthoxylum americanum

Saccharomycetaceae (Eumycota [Fungi])
Saccharomyces cerevisiae

Salicaceae
Populus x jackii
Populus tremuloides
Salix mollissima
Salix nigra
Salix purpurea
Salix triandra

Santalaceae
Okoubaka aubrevillei
Santalum album

Sapindaceae
Paullinia cupana
Paullinia pinnata

Sarraceniaceae
Sarracenia purpurea

Saururaceae
Anemopsis californica

Scrophulariaceae
Chelone glabra
Digitalis purpurea
Epifagus virginiana
Euphrasia officinalis
Gratiola officinalis
Linaria vulgaris
Scrophularia nodosa
Verbascum thapsus
Veronica beccabunga
Veronicastrum virginicum

Simaroubaceae
Ailanthus altissima
Castela erecta subsp. *texana*
Quassia amara
Simaba cedron
Simarouba amara

Smilacaceae
Smilax regelii

Solanaceae
Atropa belladonna
Brugmansia arborea
Brugmansia sanguinea
Brunfelsia uniflora
Capsicum annuum
Datura ferox
Datura metel
Datura stramonium
Fabiana imbricata
Hyoscyamus niger
Mandragora officinarum
Nicotiana tabacum
Physalis alkekengi
Scopolia carniolica
Solanum aethiopicum
Solanum americanum
Solanum capsicoides
Solanum carolinense
Solanum dulcamara
Solanum lycopersicum
Solanum mammosum
Solanum nigrum
Solanum pseudocapsicum
Solanum tuberosum
Solanum virginianum

Sterculiaceae
Ambroma augusta
Cola acuminata
Theobroma cacao

Strophariaceae (Eumycota [Fungi])
Stropharia semiglobata
Panaeolus papilionaceus
Psilocybe caerulescens

Taxaceae
Taxus baccata
Taxus brevifolia

Taxodiaceae
Sequoia sempervirens

Theaceae
Camellia sinensis

Thymelaceae
Daphne mezereum

Daphne odora
Dirca palustris

Tiliaceae
Tilia cordata

Trilliaceae
Paris quadrifolia
Trillium cernuum
Trillium erectum

Tropaeolaceae
Tropaeolum majus

Turneraceae
Turnera diffusa

Typhaceae
Typha latifolia

Ulmaceae
Celtis occidentalis
Ulmus rubra

Umbelliferae see *Apiaceae*

Urticaceae
Dendrocnide sinuata
Laportea gigas
Parietaria officinalis
Urtica urens

Ustilaginaceae (Eumycota [Fungi])
Ustilago maydis

Valerianaceae
Valeriana officinalis

Verbenaceae
Phyla scaberrima
Verbena hastata
Verbena urticifolia
Vitex agnus-castus
Vitex trifolia

Violaceae
Viola odorata
Viola tricolor

Viscaceae
Viscum album

Vitaceae
Parthenocissus quinquefolia

Xanthorrhoeaceae
Xanthorrhoea arborea

Zamiaceae
Macrozamia spiralis

Zingiberaceae
Curcuma longa
Zingiber officinale

Zygophyllaceae
Guaiacum officinale
Larrea tridentata
Tribulus terrestris

Acknowledgements

The preparation of this annotated checklist has involved many sources and help from numerous individuals and institutions. We thank all those who contributed to this work and would especially like to acknowledge the following: Alan F. Baker of *A.F and S. Baker*, Pat Baker of *Your Body Ltd.*, Joan Morgan of *Helios* and Roger Barsby of *Weleda* for providing funding for this project and without whose help this work would not have taken place; Roger van Zandvoort, for supplying the list of names from his *Complete Repertory* in electronic format and for his continuous help and support over the years; Farhad Madon, Rosemarie Rees and Mike Sadka for help with setting up the nomenclature database; Tony Scott for re-structuring the nomenclature database; David Sutton for the bibliography database; Sinead O'Hara of *The Royal London Homeopathic Hospital* for providing access to the pharmacopoeia names. For help with nomenclature we thank Charles Jarvis for checking all the Linnaean names and for helpful advice on nomenclatural problems. For help on particular groups we thank Sandy Knapp, Amanda Waterfield, Peter Roberts, Brian Spooner, Beryl Simpson, John Dransfield, Piers Trehane, Toby Pennington, Zofia Lawrence, Lisa Offord, Jennifer Bryant, Mats Wedin, William Purvis, Ian Tittley, David John, Len Ellis, Mary Gibby, Alison Paul, Caroline Whitefoord, Pat Wolseley and Norman Robson. All names were checked from the Botany and General libraries of *The Natural History Museum, The Royal Botanic Gardens, Kew* and *The Wellcome Institute*. We are especially grateful to Judith Magee, for locating elusive publications, and Malcolm Beasley, Carol Gokce, Debbie Gale and Emma-Louise Smith on other library matters. Finally special thanks to Mike Gilbert for advice on the final editing.

References cited

Allen, T.F. 1874-79. *Encyclopedia of Pure Materia Medica.* 11 volumes. Boericke and Tafel. Philadelphia.

Barthel, H. & Klunker, W. 1987. *Synthetic Repertory.* 3rd ed. 3 volumes. New Delhi.

Boericke, W. 1927. *Pocket Manual of Homoeopathic Materia Medica.* 9th ed. Boericke & Runyon. New York.

Bridson, G.D.R. & Smith, E.R. (eds). 1991. *B-P-H/S: Botanico-Periodicum-Huntianum : Supplementum.* Hunt Institute for Botanical Documentation. Pittsburgh.

Briquet, J. 1935. *International rules of botanical nomenclature, adopted by the ... Congresses of Vienna, 1905, and Brussels, 1910, revised by the ... Congress of Cambridge, 1930 /* compiled by the Editorial Committee for Nomenclature from the report of the Subsection of Nomenclature prepared by J. Briquet. Verlag von Gustav Fischer. Jena.

Brummitt, R.K. & Powell, C.E. (eds). 1992. *Authors of Plant Names.* Royal Botanic Gardens. Kew.

Brummitt, R.K. compiled by. 1992. *Vascular Plant Families and Genera.* Royal Botanic Gardens. Kew.

CABI Bioscience. *"Database of Fungal Names -Funindex".* <http://www.speciesfungorum.org/>. [Accessed: Mar 2000 - Nov 2000]

Centre for Plant Biodiversity Research. *"Australian Plant Name Index - APNI".* <http://www.anbg.gov.au/cgi-bin/apni>. [Accessed: Oct 1999 - May 2000]

Clarke, J.H. 1900. *A Dictionary of Practical Materia Medica.* Homoeopathic Publishing Co. London.

Farjon, A. 1998. *World checklist and bibliography of conifers.* Royal Botanic Gardens. Kew.

Farr, E.R., Leussink, J.A. & Stafleu, F.A. 1979. *Index Nominum Genericorum (Plantarum).* 3 volumes. Bohn, Scheltema & Holkema. Utrecht.

Farr, E.R., Leussink, J.A. & Zijlstra, G. 1986. *Index Nominum Genericorum (Plantarum) Supplementum 1.* Bohn, Scheltema & Holkema. Utrecht.

Frodin, D.G. 1984. *Guide to Standard Floras of the World : an annotated, geographically arranged systematic bibliography of the principal floras, enumerations, checklists and chorological atlases of different areas.* Cambridge University Press. Cambridge.

German Homoeopathic Pharmacopoeia (GHP). 1990. English translation of the 1st, 1978 ed. Comprising GHP 1 1978, 1st supplement 1981, 2nd supplement 1983, 3rd supplement 1985, 4th supplement 1985. Sponsored by the British Homeopathic Association. Deutscher Apotheker Verlag. Stuttgart.

German Homoeopathic Pharmacopoeia (GHP). 1993. English translation of the 5th supplement (1991) to the 1978 ed. Sponsored by the British Homeopathic Association. Deutscher Apotheker Verlag. Stuttgart.

Ghose, S.C. 1980. *Drugs of Hindoosthan.* 8th ed. Hahnemann Publishing Co. Pvt. Ltd. Calcutta, India.

Gledhill, D. 1989. *The Names of Plants.* 2nd ed. Cambridge University Press. Cambridge.

Govaerts, R., Frodin, D.G. & Radcliffe-Smith, A. 2000. *World checklist and bibliography of Euphorbiaceae (with Pandaceae) : Introduction; Euphorbiaceae: general references; Euphorbiaceae: Aalius-Crossophora 1.* Royal Botanic Gardens. Kew.

Govaerts, R., Frodin, D.G. & Radcliffe-Smith, A. 2000. *World checklist and bibliography of Euphorbiaceae (with Pandaceae) : Euphorbiaceae: Croton-Excoecariopsis 2.* Royal Botanic Gardens. Kew.

Govaerts, R., Frodin, D.G. & Radcliffe-Smith, A. 2000. *World checklist and bibliography of Euphorbiaceae (with Pandaceae) : Fahrenheitia-Oxydectes 3.* Royal Botanic Gardens. Kew.

Govaerts, R., Frodin, D.G. & Radcliffe-Smith, A. 2000. *World checklist and bibliography of Euphorbiaceae (with Pandaceae) : Euphorbiaceae: Pachystemon-Zygospermum; Pandaceae; Doubtful and excluded names and taxa 4.* Royal Botanic Gardens. Kew.

Govaerts, R. & Frodin, D.G. 1998. *World checklist and bibliography of Fagales (Betulaceae, Corylaceae, Fagaceae and Ticodendraceae).* Royal Botanic Gardens. Kew.

Govaerts, R. & Frodin, D.G. 1996. *World checklist and bibliography of Magnoliaceae.* Royal Botanic Gardens. Kew.

Greuter, W. et al. 2000. *International Code of Botanical Nomenclature (Saint Louis Code) : adopted by the Sixteenth International Botanical Congress, St Louis, Missouri July-August 1999.* Koeltz Scientific Books. Königstein, Germany.

Hahnemann, S. 1880-81. *Materia Medica Pura.* 2 volumes. Hahnemann Publishing Society. London.

Hale, E.M. 1875. *Materia Medica of the New Remedies.* 4th ed. Boericke and Tafel. Philadelphia.

Hawksworth, D.L., Kirk, P.M., Sutton, B.C. & Pegler, D.N. 1995. *Ainsworth & Bisby's Dictionary Of The Fungi.* 8th ed. CAB International. Wallingford, Oxfordshire.

Hering, C. 1879-91. *Guiding Symptoms of Our Materia Medica.* 10 volumes. American Homoeopathic Publishing Society. Philadelphia.

Heywood, V.H. (ed.). 1978. *Flowering Plants of the World.* Oxford University

Press. Oxford.

IK: Index Kewensis. 2.0. 1997. *CD-ROM.* Oxford University Press. Oxford.

Information on California plants for education, research and conservation. *"CalFlora".* <http://elib.cs.berkeley.edu/calflora/>. [Accessed: Jan 2000 - Oct 2000]

Jeffrey, C. 1973. *Biological Nomenclature.* Edward Arnold (Publishers) Ltd. London.

Julian, O. 1979. *Materia Medica of New Homoeopathic Remedies.* Beaconsfield Publishers Ltd. Beaconsfield.

Kent, J.T. 1957. *Repertory of the Homoeopathic Materia Medica.* 6th ed. Ehrhart & Karl. Chicago.

Knerr, C.B. 1951. *A Repertory of Hering's guiding symptoms of our materia medica.* 3rd ed. M. Bhattacharya. Calcutta.

Lawrence G.H.M., Buchheim, A.F.G., Daniels, G.S., & Dolezal, H. 1968. *B-P-H: Botanico-Periodicum-Huntianum.* Hunt Botanical Library. Pittsburgh.

Legume Web. *"International Legume Database & Information Service - ILDIS", version 4.10 & 4.20.* <http://www.ildis.org/LegumeWeb/>. [Accessed: Oct 1999 - Sept 2000]

Leyel, C.F. (ed.). 1992. *Grieve - A Modern Herbal : the medicinal, culinary, cosmetic and economic properties, cultivation and folklore of herbs, grasses, fungi, shrubs and trees with all their modern scientific uses.* .Tiger Books International. London.

Linnaeus, C. 1749. *Materia Medica.* Stockholm.

Mabberley, D.J. 1997. *The Plant Book : a portable dictionary of the vascular plants.* 2nd ed. Cambridge University Press. Cambridge.

Manilal, K.S. (ed.). 1980. *The Botany and History of Hortus Malabaricus.* Balkema. Rotterdam.

Mennega, E.A. & Stafleu, F.A. 1992. *Taxonomic literature : a selective guide to botanical publications and collections with dates, commentaries and types.* Supplement 1 A-Ba. Koeltz Scientific Books. Königstein, Germany.

Mennega, E.A. & Stafleu, F.A. 1993. *Taxonomic literature : a selective guide to botanical publications and collections with dates, commentaries and types.* Supplement 2 Be-Bo. Koeltz Scientific Books. Königstein, Germany.

Mennega, E.A. & Stafleu, F.A. 1995. *Taxonomic literature : a selective guide to botanical publications and collections with dates, commentaries and types.* Supplement 3 Br-Ca. Koeltz Scientific Books. Königstein, Germany.

Mennega, E.A. & Stafleu, F.A. 1997. *Taxonomic literature : a selective guide to botanical publications and collections with dates, commentaries and types.* Supplement 4 Ce-Cz. Koeltz Scientific Books. Königstein, Germany.

Mennega, E.A. & Stafleu, F.A. 1998. *Taxonomic literature : a selective guide to botanical publications and collections with dates, commentaries and types.* Supplement 5 Da-Di. Koeltz Scientific Books. Königstein, Germany.

Mennega, E.A. & Stafleu, F.A. 2000. *Taxonomic literature : a selective guide to botanical publications and collections with dates, commentaries and types.* Supplement 6 Do-E. Koeltz Scientific Books. Königstein, Germany.

Millspaugh, C.F. 1892. *Medicinal Plants : an illustrated descriptive guide to plants indigenous to and naturalized in the United States which are used in medicine.* 2 volumes. John C. Yorston & Co. Philadelphia.

Ministry of Health – The French republic. 1991. *French Pharmacopoeia (English translation).* 10th ed. 6th supplement. L'adrapharm. Paris.

Missouri Botanical Garden. *"w3TROPICOS"*. <http://mobot.mobot.org/W3T/Search/pick.html>. [Accessed: Oct 1999-Oct 2000]

Missouri Botanical Garden. *"Flora of Panama Checklist "*. <http://mobot.mobot.org/W3T/Search/panama.html>. [Accessed: Oct 1999 - Oct 2000]

Missouri Botanical Garden. *"Peru Checklist"*. <http://mobot.mobot.org/W3T/Search/peru.html>. [Accessed: Jan 2000 - Sept 2000]

Missouri Botanical Garden. *"Flora Mesoamericana: Lista Anotada - w3FM"*. <http://mobot.mobot.org/W3T/Search/meso.html>. [Accessed: Oct 1999 - Oct 2000]

Missouri Botanical Garden. *"Flora of China Checklist - FCC"*. <http://mobot.mobot.org/W3T/Search/foc.html>. [Accessed: Oct 1999 - Oct 2000]

Morton, J.F. 1931. *Atlas of medicinal plants of Middle America : Bahamas to Yucatan.* Charles C. Thomas. Springfield.

Saccardo, P.A. 1883-1911. *Sylloge Fungorum Omnium Hucusque Cognitorum.* Patavia.

Schroyens, F. 1993-94. *Blueprint for a New Repertory: Synthesis.* 5.2 ed. Homeopathic Book Publishers. London.

Simpson, B.B. & Ogorzaly, M.C. 1995. *Economic botany : plants in our world.*.2nd ed. McGraw-Hill. New York, London.

Singer, R. 1986. *The Agaricales in Modern Taxonomy.* 4th ed. Koenigstein. Koeltz.

Stace, C.A. 1997. *New flora of the British Isles, with illustrations mainly by Hilli Thompson..* 2nd ed. Cambridge University Press. Cambridge.

Stace, C.A. 1953. *Taxon* **2**: 37-62, *Species Plantarum 1753 - 1 May - 1953.* International Bureau for Plant Taxonomy and Nomenclature. Utrecht,

Netherlands.

Stafleu, F.A. 1967. *Taxonomic Literature. A selective guide to botanical publications with dates, commentaries and types.(= Regnum Vegetabile Vol. 52).* International Bureau for Plant Taxonomy and Nomenclature. Utrecht.

Stafleu, F.A. & Cowan, R.S. 1976-88. *Taxonomic literature : a selective guide to botanical publications and collections with dates, commentaries and types.* 2nd ed. 7 volumes. Bohn, Scheltema & Holkema. Utrecht, Netherlands.

Stearn, W.T. 1992. *Botanical Latin : history, grammar, syntax, terminology and vocabulary.* 4th ed. David & Charles. London.

Tavole di Botanica sistematica. *"Funghi indice".* <http://www.dipbot.unict.it/sistematica/Funghind.html>. [Accessed: Nov 2000]

The Boletes of California. *"Species Index".* <http://www.mykoweb.com/boletes/>. [Accessed: Aug 2000]

The Committee on Pharmacopoeia of the American Institute of Homoeopathy. 1964. *The Homoeopathic Pharmacopoeia of the United States. Revised.* 7th ed. Boericke & Tafel. Philadelphia

The Plant Names Project 1999. *"International Plant Names Index - IPNI".* <http://www.ipni.org/searches/query_ipni.shtml>. [Accessed: Jan 2000 - Sept 2000]

Tutin, T.G. et al. (eds). 1964-80. *Flora Europaea.* 5 volumes. Cambridge University Press. Cambridge.

van Zandvoort, R. 1994-96. *The Complete Repertory : Mind - Generalities.* Institute for Research in Homeopathic Information and Symptomatology. The Netherlands.